Kale & Kravings

Nourishing Dorm Room Recipes & Wellness Practices for Students

By Sloane Elizabeth

KALE & KRAVINGS:
NOURISHING DORM ROOM PRACTICES & WELLNESS PRACTICES FOR STUDENTS.
© 2018 by Kale & Kravings. All rights reserved.
www.kaleandkravings.com
Cover & book design by Pilar O'Connor
Food styling & photography by Sloane Elizabeth
ISBN: 978-0-578-52256-2

Table of Contents

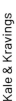
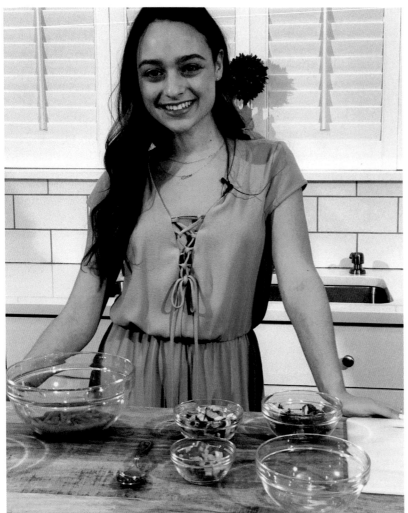

HI! I'M KALE

Hi! My name is Sloane Elizabeth, but you can call me "Kale." As a college student (and a wellness coach, Instagram influencer, foodie, chef, fitness fanatic, and admirer of all things health & wellness), I understand the struggle of balancing good grades, a thriving social life, a well-rested body, and meaningful relationships, all while slowly dragging my slightly hungover self to a 9 a.m. lecture every Friday morning, green smoothie in hand. College is known to be "the best 4 years of our lives"...but it's also characterized by unhealthy habits like late night greasy pizza, drunken nights out, sleepless hours of studying (or cramming if we're being real), and frequent trips to the student health center. I, for one, refuse to accept these conditions bestowed upon us as 18-22 year olds...why should we have to choose between wild fun or healthy safe seclusion? We should (and can) have both! That is why I have decided to put together this guide to show you how to balance college life as best as I know how : K&K style.

Before we go any further, I want to acknowledge that I am nowhere near perfect, nor am I a professional. I only speak from my own research, experience, and education on the matters enclosed in this book. So, why should you trust me? That's a good question, so let's get to know each other a bit better...

My health and wellness journey is far from your average weight loss, sports injury, or struggling celiac story. Rather, I was a Varsity cheerleader and dancer from Los Angeles who owned a baking business. Yep – real butter, lots of gluten, and tons of sugar filled my grocery cart daily. I had always taken my health and slim figure for granted; I had "good genes," as they say. I also had a huge sweet tooth; the dreamy smell of melting butter and hypnotizing vision of my pink KitchenAid mixer danced through my head as I sat in an AP Physics class that I didn't understand. (Thankfully, I'll never have to take college level Physics!)

As I neared the end of high school, I began to notice that I had hips and a few curves that weren't there before, and that maybe I couldn't eat 5 cookie-layered brownies a day

and still feel energized and healthy. Living in LA, there was no shortage of resources for girls looking to get "healthier" and "slimmer" or to find that "natural, no-makeup glow," so I started reading and researching how to be "healthy." I never believed every magazine article or diet food label that claimed "10 pounds gone in 5 days". "The slimming juice cleanse" was not for me, nor was the "magic weight management pill." Instead, I dug deeper, and read scientific journals and nutrition studies. I started making small changes to my diet – more veggies, less processed food – but I wanted to know more.

Entering college, I brought with me a healthy mindset – I would eat the food on the meal plan, buy healthy snacks, and bring my own avocado to the dining hall for breakfast (because avocado toast, duh!). But a year of late night cookies, southern inspired dinners, and lots of academic stress later, I returned home bearing exhaustion and illness. It finally hit me that the food we eat is a direct reflection of our performance – athletically, mentally, and physically. I realized that there was real science behind nutrition and the biological pathways responsible for breaking down and absorbing different nutrients, and I was hungry to understand it all.

Sloane Elizabeth

On May 16, 2016, I created my Instagram account, Kale & Kravings.

My approach to healthy living in college and at home has shifted a lot since that summer of 2016. At first, I was all about making "rules" that would inevitably get broken – focus on protein and veggies, limit carbs, dessert only twice a week. The more I learned through books and documentaries, the more rules I added: cut out most animal products, minimize fruit, decrease carbs, reintroduce more animal protein...it was a never ending cycle of desperately trying to figure out how to be healthy the "right way." Finally, I was introduced to holistic health – the concept that has brought me the most peace, fulfillment, and happiness since starting Kale & Kravings. My focus continues to be geared towards wellness – feeling full, whole, and authentically my best self...and that is exactly what I hope to convey in my approach to healthy college living. As you will learn, being healthy is about SO much more than the food on our plates, and in what follows you will find the tools you need to start (or continue) a life of health and wellness in college, and beyond.

xo
Kale

P.S. Almost all of the photos used in this book were taken by me, on my phone, in a dorm room. They aren't fancy, because dorm room cooking isn't either! I want these recipes and resources to be accessible and easy for you to use. If I can make them in a dorm room, then you can too!

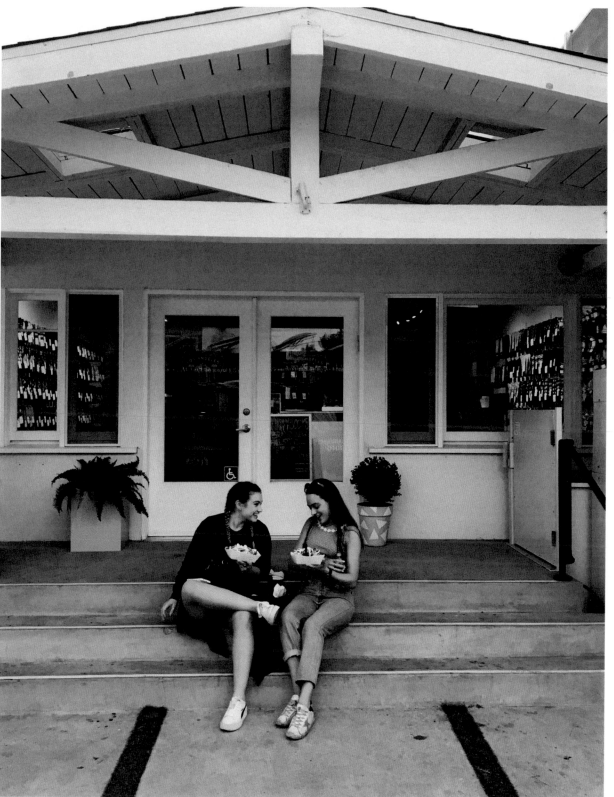

Sloane Elizabeth

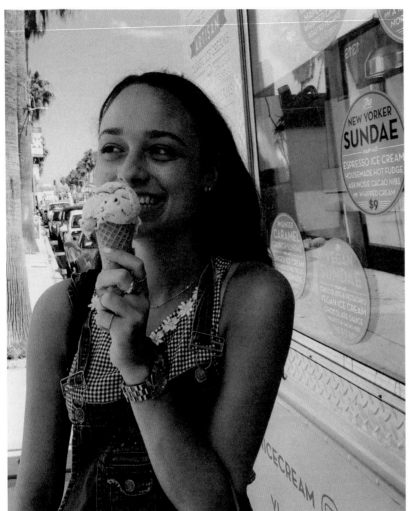

BALANCE

The term "balance" has become a buzzword within the online health and wellness community, just like the beloved words "kale," "gluten-free," "organic," and "chia seeds." While I have discussed said "balance" on my Instagram, I personally prefer the term "life." "Life" is eating 2 pieces of amazingly delicious chocolate cake at your friend's birthday celebration. "Life" is working out consistently and then not getting to the gym once during exam week. "Life" is eating chips and crackers in a foreign country when there is no fresh produce in sight. "Life" is nourishing your body with fruits and veggies all day and having a restful night of sleep. My point is that, in assuming there is a perfect balance you must strike to be healthy (i.e. the 80/20 rule, only eating dessert on the weekends, or limiting yourself to one alcoholic beverage), you are still playing by "rules" that simply do not exist. As much as I used to wish there were, there are no

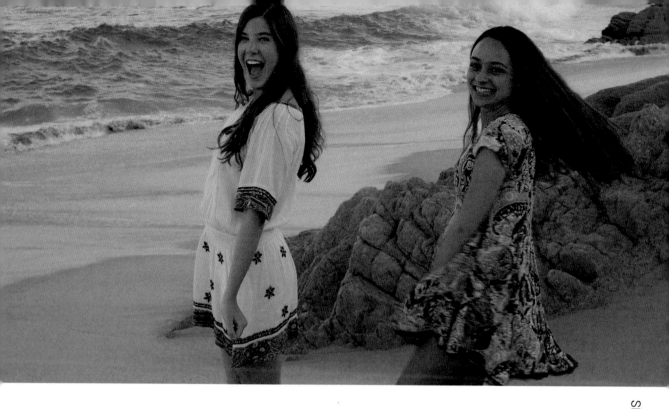

commandments instructing us on what, when, and how much to eat so that we feel our absolute best. The closest thing I can find to this is the famous phrase by Michael Pollan (author, professor, and creator of Food Inc.): "Eat food, not too much, mostly plants." I believe that living a healthy life stems from feeling happy, nourished, energized, and fulfilled in mind, body, and soul. Therefore, it is up to each individual to listen to his or her body (more on intuitive eating later) and have enough respect for that body to choose the foods, people, and activities that will best nourish the entire being. Green smoothies energize my cells every morning and fuel my workouts; yoga and meditation soothe my mind and

muscles; warm brownies with vanilla ice cream light up my soul and relationships... in this way, there is room for everything in this abundant life that we live, and nothing should be categorized as strictly "bad," "forbidden," or "restricted." It's all simply a part of life!

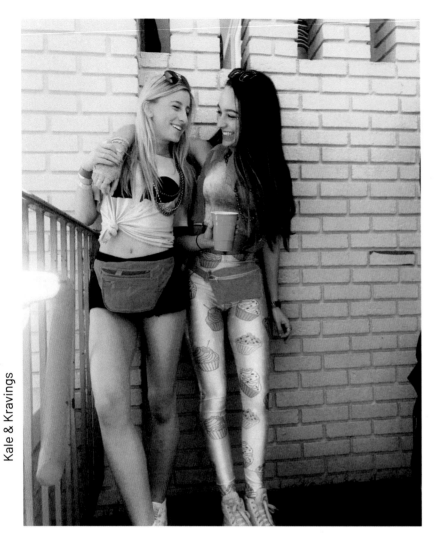

ALCOHOL

Some of my most fun memories in college include: the "Freshman only" party where we all wore yoga attire, hanging out with friends on pontoon boats, Mardi Gras weekend, and visiting friends across the country each summer. While these are not all of my favorite memories in college, they definitely place in the top 15. And what do they all have in common besides being amazing, fond memories? ALCOHOL. To some extent, alcohol and college go hand in hand. As stereotypical as it might be, parties, drugs, tailgates, and Greek life are all associated with the image of college today. I'm here to say that I've witnessed all of this in my college career. Alcohol is by no means necessary to ensure a fun time in college. It is also illegal for consumption by anyone below the age of 21...but this book is about honesty and reality, and you and I have already decided to be friends, so let's talk about it! Alcohol is, unfortunately, not "healthy" – it does not nourish our cells... in fact it is toxic to our systems. I don't believe that tequila is healthier than vodka or clear is better than amber. While these comparisons may be true, alcohol is simply a part of many healthy people's lives! I try to focus my attention on how to have the most safe and fun experience with alcohol possible while making small choices that help my body (*cough* hangover) the next day. Below are my top tips to help you make it to your 8 a.m. class after a night out:

Before:

1. EAT! Whatever you do before you drink, make sure eating is at the top of your to-do list. Healthy fats and protein will help your body slow down the metabolism pathways of your spirit of choice, but I would rather you eat a bowl of carbs than nothing at all. Please don't skip meals to "save your calories for alcohol" – drinking on an empty stomach is a recipe for disaster. You want to have fun, so you may as well indulge and enjoy the night and avoid being taken home by your friend before midnight has even struck.

2. HYDRATE! Drinking (and dancing and sweating) dehydrates your body, which can contribute to lethargy and a mean headache when you wake up the next morning. Since we all know no one actually drinks a glass

of water with every shot of vodka they take, do yourself a favor and load up on that H2O beforehand.

During:

1. BEWARE OF SUGAR! Mixed drinks can taste seemingly free of alcohol if they're concocted with soda, fruit juice, and bubbly water. While some may view this as a positive, it is also a sure way to end up drunker and more hungover than you anticipated. I believe that mixing and chasing drinks with the classic sugar-filled drinks (sodas, juice, margarita mixes) is the top cause of a hangover...instead, opt for sugar-free alternatives (Vitamin Water Zero, La Croix, bubbly water with lime) to keep that hangover at bay.

2. WATER! I know we said we wouldn't, but if you're an angel, drink water while you're out. Especially if you're hot and sweaty from dancing up a storm!

Sloane Elizabeth

11

After:

1. WATER! Here we are again with our dear friend H2O... definitely drink a couple of glasses of water before you hit the sack. Don't force yourself to guzzle down a full liter (like I used to) because that can be quite taxing on your digestive system and bladder. Definitely keep a bottle of water by your bed though...you'll thank yourself when you wake up.

2. DRIVE BY THE FAST FOOD! Drunk eating tastes so good in the moment, and I know how appetizing those burgers/fries/hotdogs/quesadillas/nachos sound in the moment. Do what you will (#life), but know that your stomach probably won't be too thrilled with you in the morning.

3. BREAKFAST! Replenish yourself with nutrients when you wake up. If you're feeling queasy, opt for foods that are easy to digest (smoothie, plain oatmeal). Again, don't try to "make up" for the calories that you drank last night by not eating. You went out, hopefully had fun, and now it's time to get back to your day!

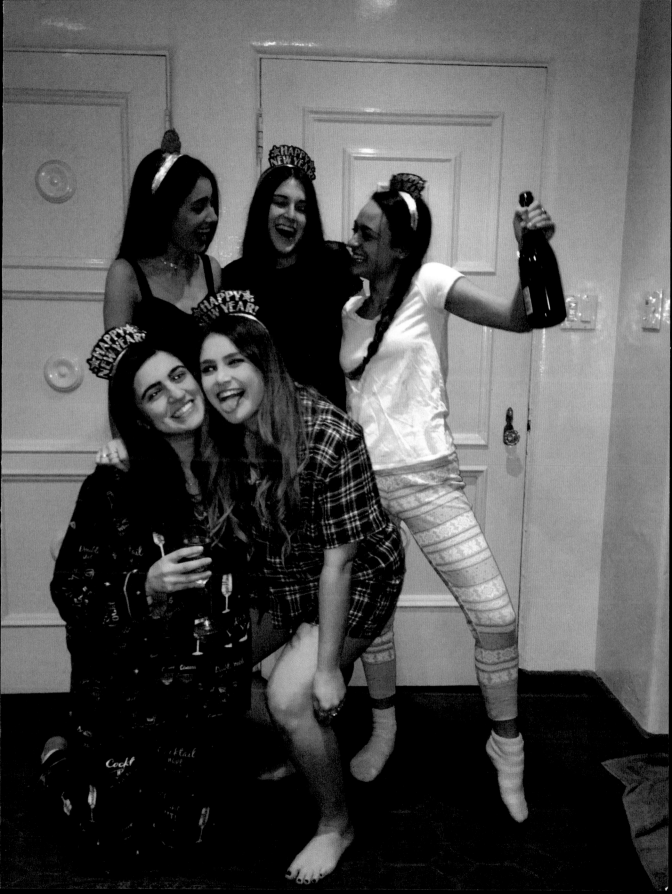

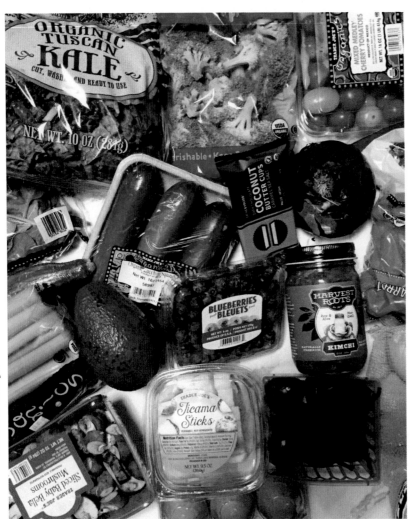

SHOPPING LIST

This guide is meant to show you how to be well and healthy while in college (and beyond), understanding that you may not have a full-size kitchen and health food store at your disposal. Here are the tools that I recommend to keep in your dorm room – they are minimal, multi-functional, and have proved to be essential in my pursuits as a dorm-room chef:

1. Mini-fridge (preferably with a freezer)
2. Microwave
3. Mini blender
4. Knife and cutting board
5. Large microwaveable bowl
6. Utensils, plates, bowls (reusable or plastic)

I also intend for this guide to be used alongside any campus meal plan you may be on. Although each school is different, I was able to use my meal plan and supplement with trips to the grocery store every few weeks. If your schedule and budget allow for this too, here is my go-to grocery list – all essentials that are used in this book:

Fruit
-Bananas
-Berries
-Avocados
-Apples
-Lemons

Vegetables
-Kale
-Romaine
-Spinach
-Carrots
-Cucumber
-Celery
-Broccoli
-Cauliflower
-Zucchini
-Cabbage
-Jicama
-Bell peppers
-Tomatoes
-Butternut squash

Spices & Herbs & Condiments
-Cinnamon
-Black pepper
-Pink sea salt
-Turmeric
-Garlic
-Italian seasonings blend
-Honey (preferably Manuka honey)
-Mustard
-Avocado oil
-Kimchi
-Sauerkraut
-Tomato sauce
-Parsley

Nuts & Seeds
-Nut milk
-Nut/coconut yogurt
-Raw cashews
-Pumpkin seeds
-Sunflower seeds
-Chia seeds
-Flax seeds
-Hemp seeds
-Nut butters (preferably raw and organic, or whatever fits your budget!)

Grains & Legumes & Proteins
-Brown rice (dry or frozen)
-Quinoa (dry or frozen)
-Black beans
-Chickpeas
-Pasta
-Frozen veggie burgers
-Eggs (preferably organic, pasture-raised, or whatever fits your budget!)

Sloane Elizabeth

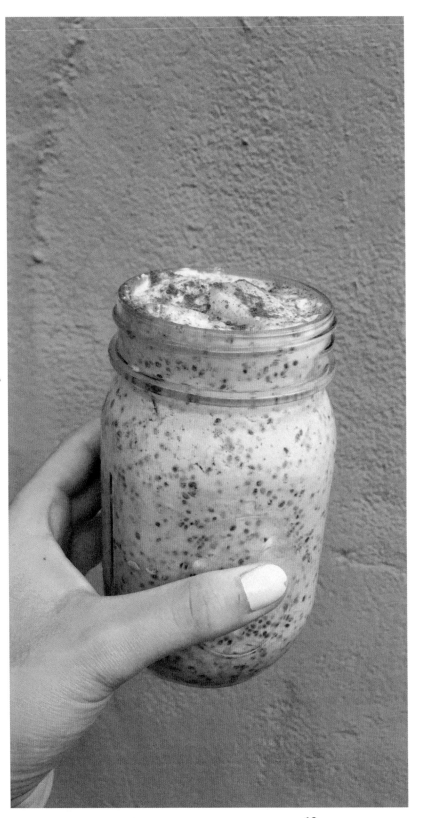

BREAKFAST RECIPES

Scrambled Eggs

Ingredients:

-Two Eggs
-1 Cup chopped veggies:tomatoes, bell peppers, broccoli, mushrooms
-Handful of spinach
-Pepper + salt

Directions:

-Crack two eggs into a microwave safe bowl (paperor plastic). Whisk the eggs together with pepper & salt.
-Add the chopped veggies and spinach to the bowl and mix the contents.
-Microwave for one minute.
-Remove the bowl from the microwave and mix the contents again with a fork to "re-scramble" the eggs.
-Microwave for another two minutes.
-Continue to microwave and "re-scramble" until the eggs and veggies are thoroughly cooked through (usually around 2.5 minutes).

Sloane Elizabeth

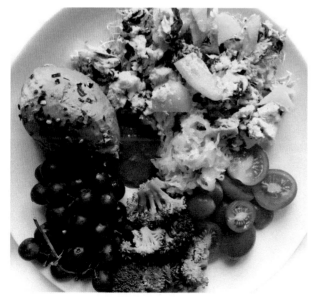

Overnight Oats:

Ingredients:

-1/3 Cup rolled oats

-½ Cup unsweetened almond milk

-½ Scoop vanilla protein powder

-2 Tbsp chia seeds

-¼ Tsp cinnamon

-1/3 Cup dairy-free yogurt (optional)

-Optional Toppings: berries, nut butter, granola, mixed nuts, coconut

-Optional add ins: ½ apple (grated), ½ zucchini (grated), ½ tsp matcha powder

Directions:

-Mix all of the ingredients in a bowl or container.

-Refrigerate overnight, add toppings, and enjoy!

Suggested flavor combos:

Green Machine:

-Base + ½ zucchini, shredded + 1 tsp matcha

Berry:

-Base + 1 tsp acai powder

-Toppings: ¼ cup mixed berries + 2 tbs peanut/ almond butter + 1 tbsp goji berries

Apple pie:

-Base + 1 apple, chopped or shredded + pinch of nutmeg

-Toppings: ¼ cup chopped walnuts + dairy free yogurt

-Base + ½ scoop chocolate protein powder + 2 tsp cacao powder + cacao nibs

-Toppings: ½ sliced banana + 2 tbsp peanut butter

Kale & Kravings

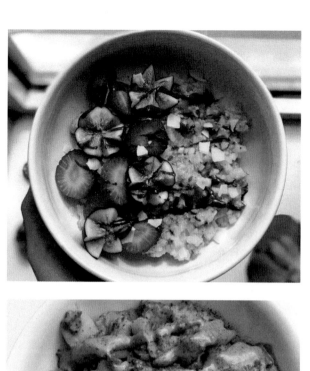
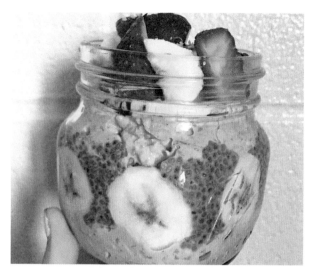

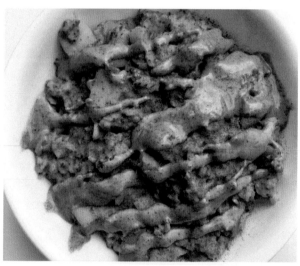
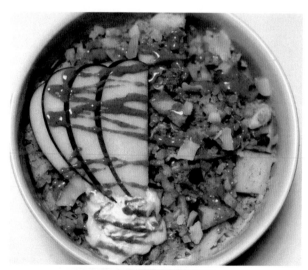

Sloane Elizabeth

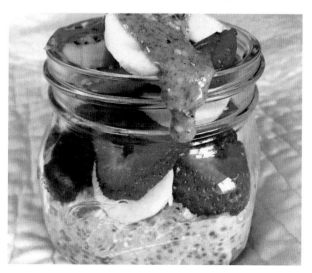
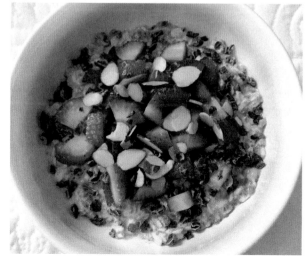

Veggie Oats:

Ingredients:
- ¼ Cup rolled oats
- 1/2 Cup cauliflower "rice"
- 1/3 Cup water or unsweetened almond milk
- 1 Tbsp chia seeds
- ¼ Tsp cinnamon
- ¼ Tsp vanilla extract
- Optional add ins: ¼ cup pumpkin, 1 apple (chopped), ¼ cup frozen berries
- Optional Toppings: berries, nut butter, granola, mixed nuts, coconut

Directions:
- Combine all ingredients in a microwave-safe bowl (make sure it is deep enough to avoid overflowing while cooking).
- Microwave for 2-4 minutes, depending on the time indicated on the oatmeal packaging.
- Remove from the microwave and stir. Continue to microwave and stir until all of the water is absorbed.
- Add toppings and enjoy!

Suggested flavor combos:

Pumpkin Pie:
- Base + ½ cup pumpkin puree + pinch of pumpkin pie spice
- Toppings: blueberries + Slivered almonds + dairy free yogurt

Berry bliss:
- Base + ½ cup frozen berries
- Toppings: 1 tbsp goji berries + 2 tbsp peanut/almond butter

Apple Pie:
- Base + 1 chopped apple + nutmeg
- Toppings: 1 tbsp almond butter + 1 tbsp unsweetened shredded coconut

Chocolate Chip Banana Bread:
- Base + 2 tsp cacao powder + ½ mashed bananas
- Toppings: 2 tbsp peanut butter

Kale & Kravings

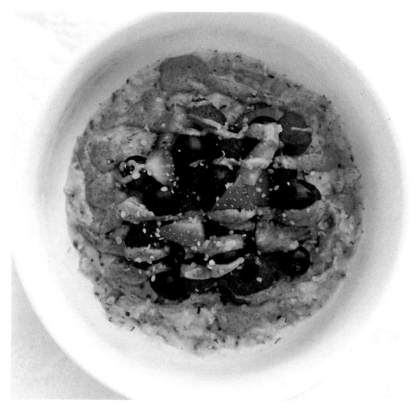

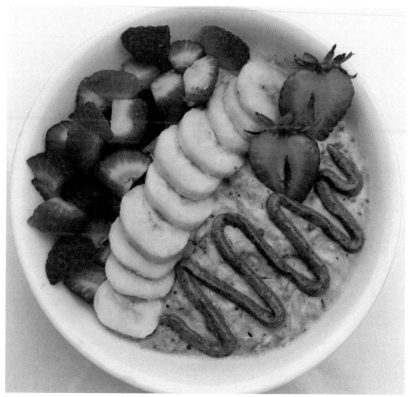

Breakfast Tacos:

Ingredients:

-2 Eggs

-2 Tortillas (corn or grainfree)

-½ Cup chopped bell peppers and mushrooms

-Handful of spinach

-Black pepper + salt

-¼ cup black beans

-Optional toppings:

salsa, ¼ avocado, hot sauce, nutritional yeast

Directions:

-Cook the 2 eggs as described in the Scrambled Eggs recipe (page 17).

-Wrap the tortillas in a damp paper towel and microwave for 15 seconds.

-Assemble the tacos: tortilla + spinach + beans + eggs + veggies + spices + toppings.

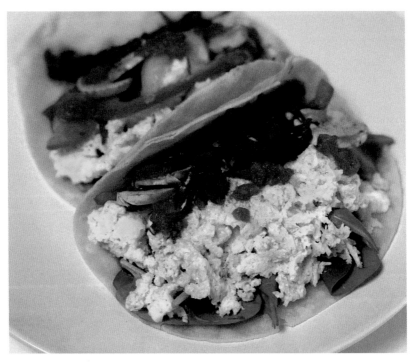

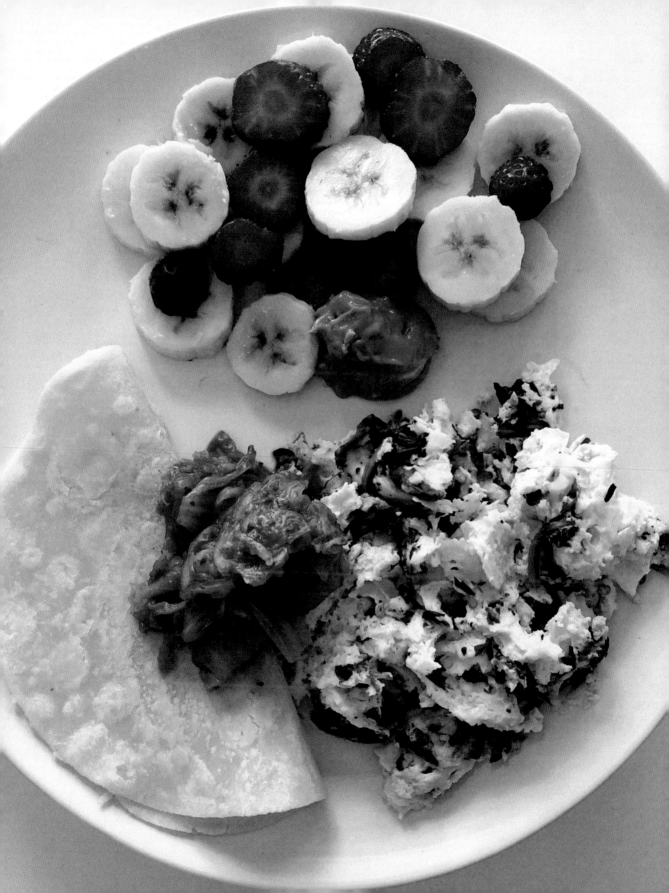

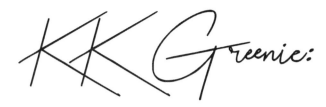

KK Greenie:

Ingredients:
-¼ Cup fruit – berries, figs, apple, banana
(use ¼ cup steamed then frozen butternut squash for a fruit-free option)
-2 Stalks of celery
-Small handful of parsley
-1.5 Cups greens – romaine, spinach, kale
-½ Tsp cinnamon
-1 Tbsp chia seeds
-1 Tbsp flax seeds
-1 Scoop vanilla protein powder
-¼ Avocado or 1 tbsp nut butter
-1 Tbsp MCT oil/coconut oil
-Water/unsweetened almond milk to blend
-Optional (but recommended) Add-Ins: 1 scoop marine collagen, 1 tsp maca powder, ½ tsp matcha, 1 tsp spirulina, 1 tbsp goji berries, 1 tsp cacao nibs, 10 drops liquid chlorophyll
-Optional Toppings: 1 tbsp bee pollen, 1 tsp pumpkin seeds, dairy-free yogurt

Directions:
-Add all ingredients to a blender. Add enough liquid to blend until smooth.
-Top and enjoy!
-Can also be made the night before and stored in a sealed container overnight in the refrigerator.

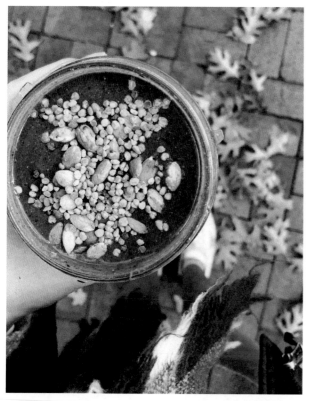

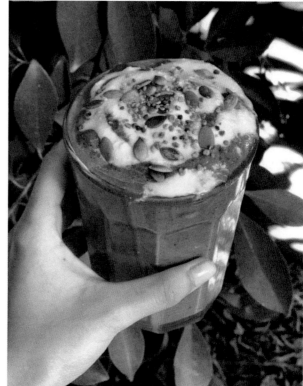

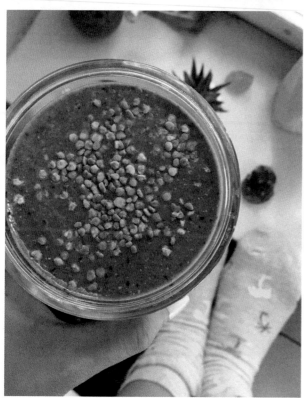

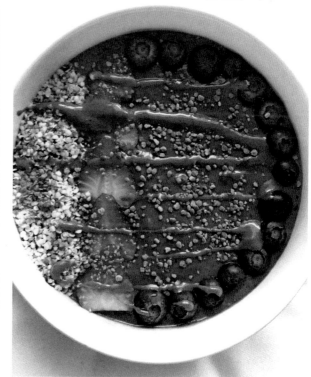

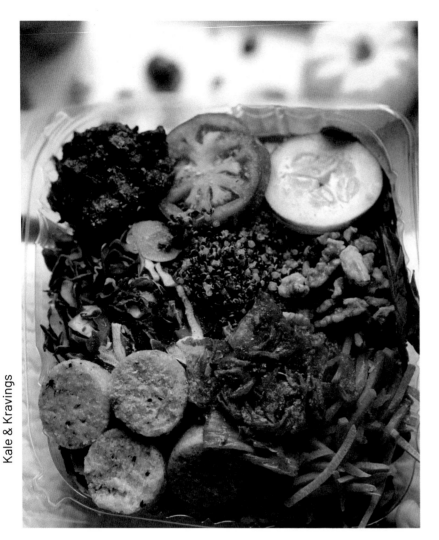

Kale & Kravings

MEAL PLANS

Let's face it...college meal plans are no gourmet, 5-star experience. Almost all college students spend their first year or two (or three if you go to school with me!) eating in a dining hall of some sort. Eating on a meal plan can be tricky for a multitude of reasons – the food can taste BAD, there may not be options that you enjoy, you don't know the source of the food, it probably isn't organic, you don't know the specific ingredients...lots of uncertainty! BUT you

should not feel hopeless, as eating on a college meal plan can be healthy, yummy, and nutritious.

My first tip for utilizing your college meal plan is to do some research and ask questions – your school may have online resources that show you the ingredients and nutrition facts of different meals offered. If that is the case, take a look and educate yourself on what you are putting into your body. If you can't find this type of resource on your own, ask the dining hall staff what the ingredients are or what type of oil is used in a particular dish! Never be afraid to ask questions in the pursuit of knowledge and health.

Secondly – load up on veggies! I personally do not eat much meat, but when I do eat fish and eggs, I prefer them to be organic and sustainably raised...probably not going to find that on campus! My meals usually consist of huge salads with fresh veggies, beans, healthy fat (nuts/seeds/avocado) and a few veggie sides (steamed or roasted vegetables, veggie soup, baked potatoes). Even if you do eat meat, it's never a bad idea to add some veggies – they'll bulk up your meal with fiber, nutrients, and flavor to keep you full longer so you aren't reaching for a bag of chips after your afternoon class.

In order to "cook" all the meals I love in my tiny dorm room, I need to have a fully stocked mini-fridge. Many times though, I don't have the time to go to a grocery store, so I use my dining hall to get ingredients! The salad bar has spinach and lettuce for my green smoothies, veggies to dip in hummus, and steamed vegetables to throw in my microwave pasta. The little food mart has bananas and berries for smoothies, hummus to snack on, and coconut water for mid-class hydration. Getting "ingredients" and bringing them back to your dorm to assemble into a new creation gives you a bit more control over the flavor/nutritional profile of your meal...and it's super fun to do with friends too!

Get creative! Sometimes my friends at school will sit down to lunch with me and ask where I got all of my food...they've missed a ton of good options in the dining hall and pass them by every day on the way to their "go-to" station. I always do a walk around the dining hall to check out all of my options before choosing what I'm going to eat. Here are some of my favorite creative dining hall hacks to keep my meal "K&K approved":

-Skip the packaged salad dressing and opt for lemon + olive oil + mustard or olive oil + balsamic vinegar

-Add a sweet potato to a salad for complex carbs, tons of vitamins, AND a salad dressing substitute

Sloane Elizabeth

27

-Opt for steamed veggies instead of sautéed to avoid creating an oily mess on your plate

-Add lemon to your water

-Munch on a package of raw veggies while you're in line for your main meal to alkalize your stomach and tide you over so you can slowly eat your meal once you're seating instead of scarfing it down

Lastly, do not stress out if you cannot control every ingredient that you put in your body (because I promise you, you won't be able to). It is true that you should aim to eat organic spinach, tomatoes, and strawberries...does that mean I avoid dining hall spinach, tomatoes, and strawberries? Of course not! As mentioned before, your college years probably will not be your healthiest years, but that doesn't mean that they have to be your unhealthiest. Accept the fact that you cannot control everything and realize that food is not the only thing that contributes to your health. Take advantage of the fact that you don't have to clean your own dirty dishes, keep a kitchen tidy, or spend hours at the stove prepping food. The time for that will come, so enjoy the meal plan as best as you can while you have it!

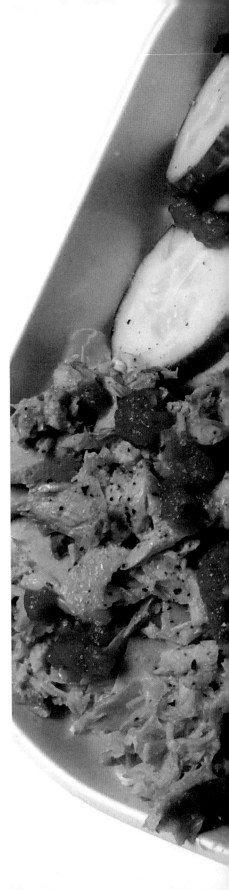

Kale & Kravings

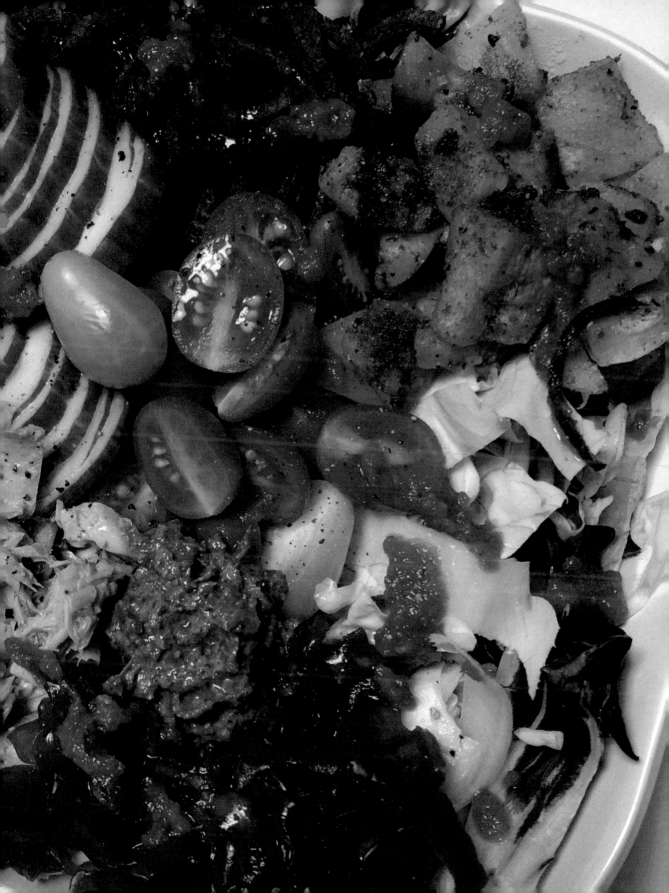

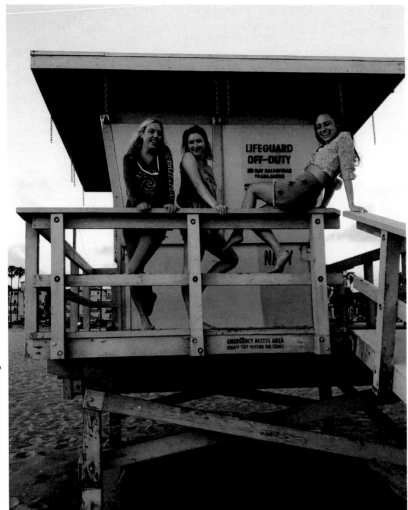

Kale & Kravings

FRIENDS

Some people are into health and wellness; some people are not. Some people workout every day; some people have never stepped foot inside a gym. Some people geek out over crystals and meditation; some people think yoga is just for hippies. Some people prioritize sleeping and studying; some people prioritize going out and socializing.

Ultimately, you will make so many friends in college (and in your life time). While some of these people may have the same priorities and passions as you, many will not.

Where health and wellness is concerned, your journey should be all about YOU. Some of your friends will also care about being healthy – they'll go to the gym, make dorm room recipes, and visit new juice bars with you. Some of your friends will support your wellness practices from afar – they may ask questions from time to time and express admiration for your dedication. Some of your friends will challenge you, lovingly poke fun at you, or genuinely not care about your health and wellness, or their own. ALL of these people have a place in your life! You don't have to exclusively surround yourself with health-conscious people to be healthy – in fact, I would advise against it! I gain so much and learn from all of my friends, especially those who challenge me and bring me back down to earth when I get too "woo-woo" with my talks of crystals, reiki, kundalini...you get the point. The most important thing about finding friends is making sure that they make you feel supported, loved, and GOOD. My foodie friends enhance my life in different ways than my super social butterfly friends or my academic and politically-minded friends. I love them all for who they are, and I know that they love me for who I am – if your friends make you feel bad about ANY of your passions, practices, or interests, they may not be a friend you want to commit a lot of time and energy to.

As many of your friends may not be into health and wellness, you may find yourself doing some activities on your own – going to workout classes, exploring farmers markets, buying new crystals, grocery shopping off campus, or trying out a meditation class.

For some, this can feel lonely and you may want to invite a friend to try out one of your cool wellness activities; or, you may be a person who loves being alone and going on adventures solo. I, myself, am an introverted extrovert (or extroverted introvert??) so I enjoy being alone, but I mostly get my energy from being with people. I find that as long as I remind myself that I should be selfish in my wellness practices and not let anyone's judgments or thoughts deter me, I am never held back or embarrassed to do all of the nutrition/fitness/spiritual activities that my heart desires! I am confident in myself, I honor my body and my interest in caring for it, and I don't press anyone to be just like me. Sometimes that does mean keeping things to myself or not sharing my love for a particular book on spirituality with a friend who I know will not be super receptive to the topic. Other times that means laughing with my friends who make fun of me for asking waiters a million question and getting everything "on the side." As long as you have a few close friends and family who DO want to hear all about your passions and dreams (non-wellness related too!), then you will never be alone. If you're struggling to find those people, then message my Instagram page and I'll listen whole-heartedly and cheer you on in any and all of your endeavors.

Sloane Elizabeth

31

One other point about friends is that you don't want to ostracize yourself or be so strict about your health that you don't let yourself relax, have fun, and LIVE a little. When a new friend asks about your health and wellness, explain to them what you do and believe, but know that they may not want to be pushed to do the same things with their body – and that is 100% fine. Mutual respect is essential to new (and old) friendships, so remember that you cannot control how other people act/eat/treat their bodies. What you can control is what YOU do. As I keep saying, college most likely will not be your healthiest years... but then again, when else do you get to live with your best friends, be a little wild, and have fun whenever you want?! SO, stick to your guns and honor your body and what it needs while also remembering that you are human, you are young, and you deserve to let loose, have 3 cookies, and wake up one morning not remembering every little detail of the night before. If you get in the habit of doing this too often where you feel like your health is suffering, then revisit your wellness intentions and some pages in this book. The point is to LIVE life in a way that makes YOU the happiest and best version of yourself. Try not to control every single aspect of your life and lead with the intention of giving yourself and the world around you all the love it deserves, whether that means getting up for an early hot yoga class or taking one more tequila shot for your friend's birthday.

Kale & Kravings

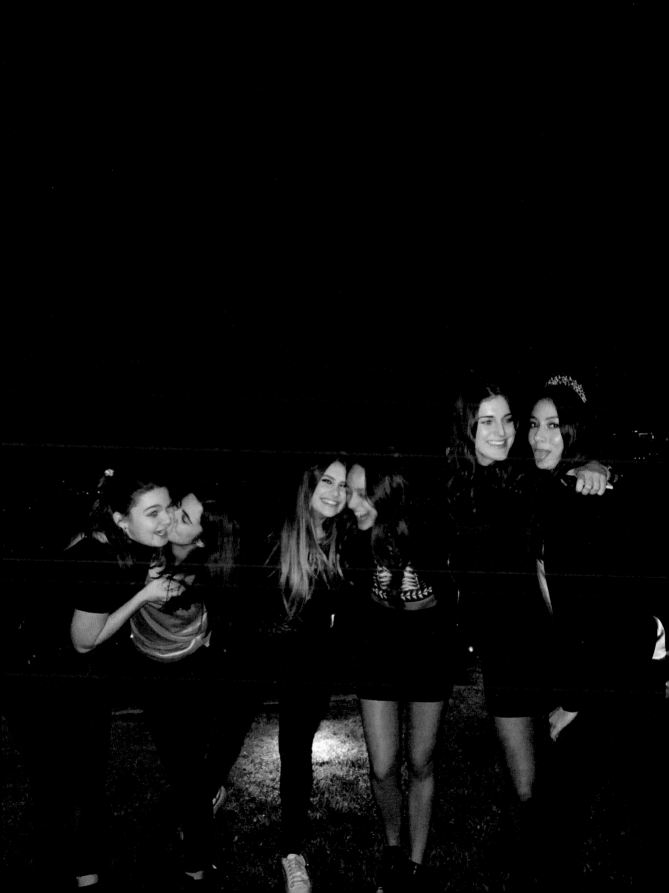

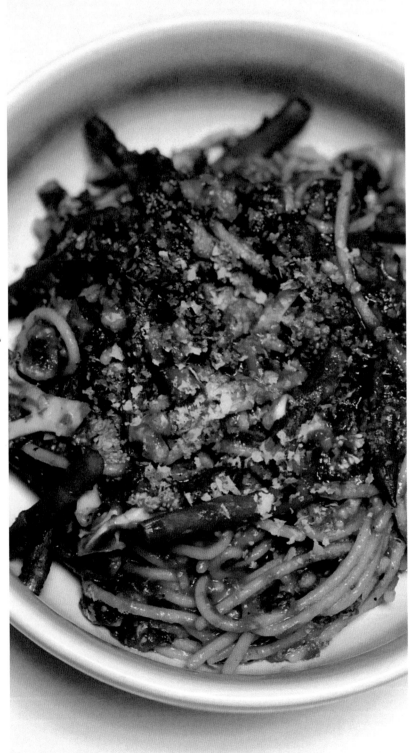

LUNCH & DINNER RECIPES

Dorm Room Pasta:

Ingredients:
-3 Oz pasta of your choice
(I prefer one made from black beans,
chickpeas, lentils, or brown rice)
-Pepper + pink salt
-Optional add-ins: tomatoes, bell peppers,
broccoli, zucchini, spinach, olives,
artichokes, avocado, mushrooms,
nutritional yeast, crushed chilli flakes
-Optional sauces: tomato sauce, vegan
pesto (page 73), lemon/garlic/olive oil

Directions:
-Put the pasta in a large,
microwave safe bowl. Add
enough water to cover the
pasta + 1 inch.
-Microwave for 6-10 minutes
(depending upon the pasta
type). Check after 6 minutes,
and continue microwaving in
2 minute increments.
-Drain the pasta and drizzle
with olive oil or avocado oil.
-Add add-ins and sauce.

Sloane Elizabeth

Suggested Flavor Combos:

-**Greek:** pasta + 1 tbsp greek salad dressing + olives + artichokes + tomatoes + steamed zucchini + avocado

-**ALL the veggies**: pasta + bolognese + steamed zucchini + steamed broccoli + spinach + mushrooms + bell peppers + olives + artichokes + nutritional yeast

-**Simple**: pasta + simple Italian + avocado + spinach + crushed chili flakes

-**Green Machine**: pasta + vegan pesto + steamed zucchini + steamed broccoli + mushrooms + avocado +nutritional yeast

Suggested sauces:

-**Vegan "Bolognese"**: tomato sauce + cooked lentils + 1 tsp crushed garlic + pepper + pink salt + ¼ cup crushed walnuts

-*Simple Italian*: olive oil + 1 tsp crushed garlic + 1/2 lemon + pepper + pink salt + crushed chili flakes

-**Vegan Pesto** (page 73)

-**Mac and Cheeze** (page 74)

-**Zucchini Alredo** (page 75)

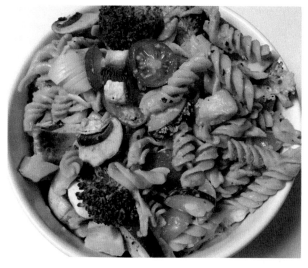 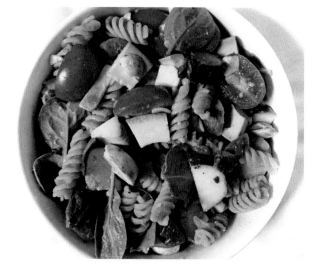

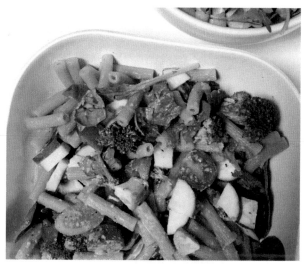 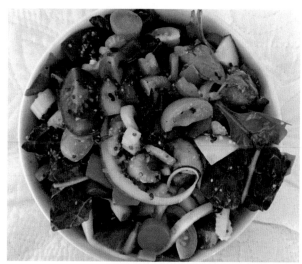

Sloane Elizabeth

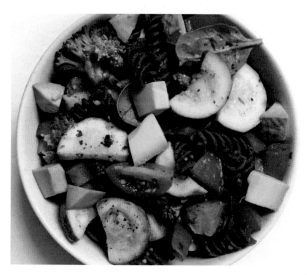 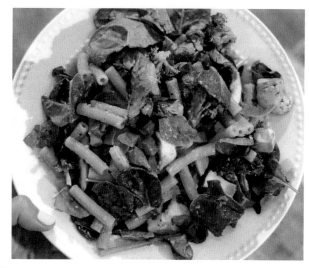

Rainbow Bowl:

Ingredients:

-Grain/Carb: quinoa, brown rice, steamed sweet potato

-Greens: arugula, butter lettuce, romaine, endive, kale, spinach, mixed greens

-Veggies: tomatoes, bell peppers, cucumber, cabbage, carrots, mushroom, jicama, artichokes, radishes

-Protein: black beans, chickpeas, lentils, hard-boiled egg, salmon, tuna, veggie burger

-Fat: avocado, olives, pumpkin seeds, walnuts, sunflower seeds, flax seeds

-Dressing: lemon, Dijon mustard, salad dressing,hummus, salsa, balsamic vinegar, apple cider vinegar

-Seasonings/Extras: pepper, pink salt, garlic, Italian seasoning, crushed chili flakes, nutritional yeast, kimchi, sauerkraut.

Directions:

-Choose 1 grain + 2 greens + unlimited veggies + 1 protein + 1 fat + 1 dressing + 3 seasonings.

-Combine in a bowl and dig in!

Kale & Kravings

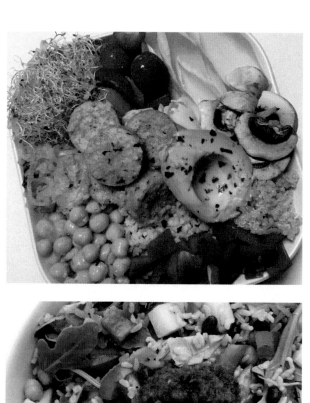 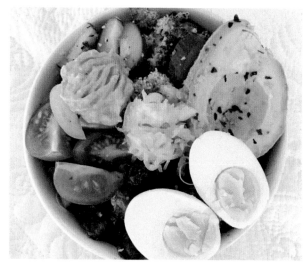

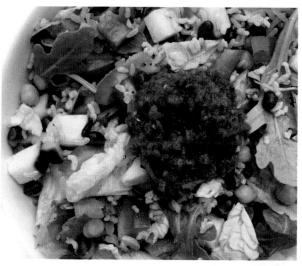 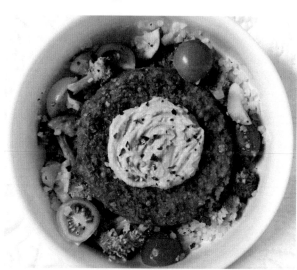

Sloane Elizabeth

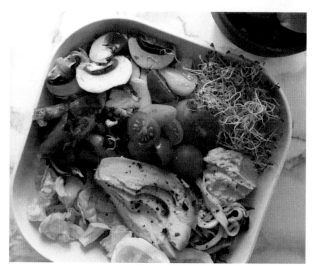 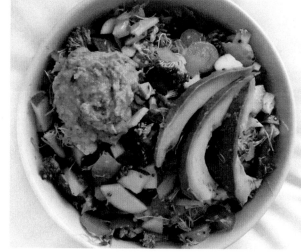

Spaghetti Squash:

Ingredients:
-1 Small Spaghetti Squash
-Sauce (tomato sauce, cheeze (page 74), or zucchini alfredo (page 75).

Directions:
-Microwave squash for 2 minutes.
-Carefully cut the squash openlength-wise.
-Scoop out the seeds.
-Place halves on a plate, flesh side down, with a bit of water.
-Microwave for 8-12 minutesuntil the flesh is tender.
-Use a fork to scrape the squash and form the "spaghetti".
-Add sauce and veggies and/or protein of choice.

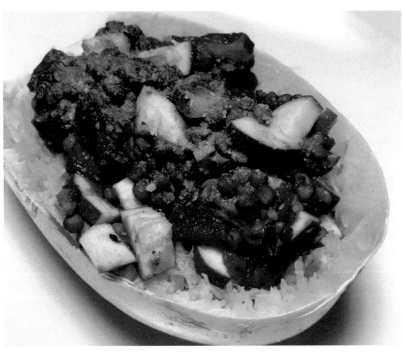

Veggie Tacos:

Ingredients:

-2 Tortillas (cor or grainfree)

-1/4 Cup hummus

-1/4 Cup lettuce

-1/2 Zucchini, sliced

-1/2 Cup cauliflower

-1 Tomato

-1/2 Avocado

-2 Tbsp nutritional yeast

-Optional spices: garlic+paprika+cumin

Directions:

-Add cauliflower, zucchini, and spices to a microwave safe bowl and cover with a damp paper towel.

-Microwave for 4 minutes until steamed thoroughly.

-Wrap the tortillas in a damp paper towel and microwave for 15 seconds.

-Assemble the tacos: tortilla + hummus + lettuce + steamed veggies + sliced tomato + avocado + nutritional yeast + pepper + pink salt.

Sloane Elizabeth

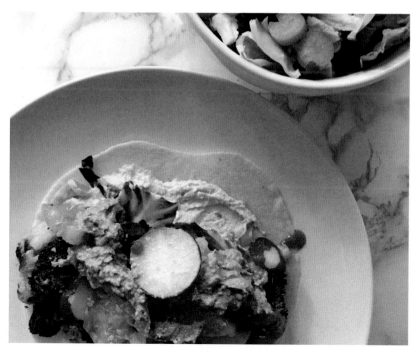

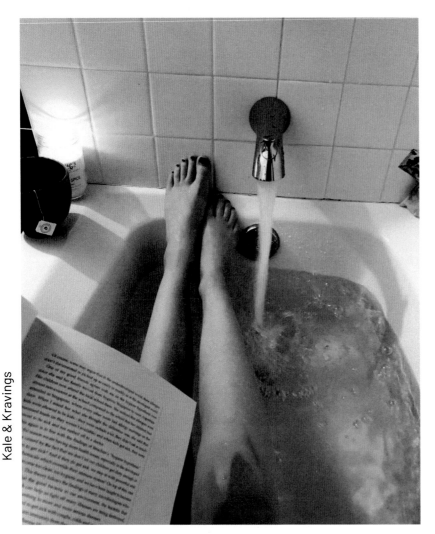

Kale & Kravings

SELF CARE

I have never been someone who enjoys lying on the couch all day binge-watching Netflix. I am most productive when I have a tight deadline, and I enjoy making long lists and crossing things off as I accomplish them. I thrive with a busy schedule, but sometimes I go overboard and find myself feeling burnt out, tired, and sick after a week or two of non-stop "go" time. In 2017, I slowly started embracing many self-care practices that I now incorporate into my daily routine.

Below are the practices that I have found, tried, and loved. You may gravitate towards one or two, or none at all...that's all fine! Experiment with different practices and find what feels best for you. All I ask is that you carve out some serious YOU time every single day away from screens. This is a time to check in with yourself, thank yourself, decompress, relax, breathe, and love every inch of you!

Meditation

I was definitely someone who was scared to try meditation. It was an intimidating task that I didn't entirely understand, and I assumed I wouldn't be "good" at it. Now, about seven months after meditating for the first time, I am completely hooked and rarely go a day without meditating. My meditations usually happen in my bed after I've just woken up for 5-10 minutes. You don't have to climb to the top of a mountain and sit alone for 10 hours to gain the benefits of meditation, nor is there one way to meditate! There are essentially no rules to meditation...except to BREATHE. The point is to be mindful, present, and relaxed. Meditation brings me mental clarity. It helps me begin my day with positivity and radiant light. It allows me to align myself with the flow of the Universe. If you are new to meditation, I recommend starting by searching for a 5 minute guided meditation online. From there, you may want to take a group meditation class at a yoga studio or find some books that will teach you more and help you deepen your spiritual practices.

Crystals

Even if crystals weren't energetically magical and they were just pretty stones, I would STILL love them! Crystals are stones from deep within the Earth's crust that radiate different energetic frequencies. These vibrations align with different chakras within our bodies in order to help enhance or release a block from your energy. They are associated with different colors, sounds, emotions, and body parts. Essentially, crystals help bring you back into alignment with yourself and the Universe. There are hundreds of different crystals

Sloane Elizabeth

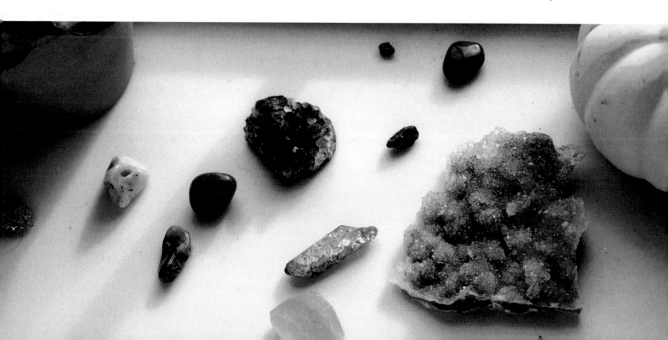

that do hundreds of different things to benefit you. Even if you don't know what a certain crystal does or you don't fully believe in their power, they will still do their job. When looking for crystals, pick the ones that you inexplicably gravitate towards. You can find crystals in spiritual shops and yoga studios around the world. Once you've chosen your crystals, you'll want to cleanse and charge them. There are many different rituals for doing this, so do a bit of research and choose the method that you like best...similar to meditation, there is no one correct way to do this. Many people charge their crystals on full moon and new moon nights. Once they are charged and ready to go, you can meditate with your crystals, hold them, look at them, carry them with you, or do nothing at all! Even if you don't charge them and cleanse them or get super into the whole crystal thing, merely having these pretty tokens of good energy will absolutely help you raise your vibrations and remind you to focus on cultivating positive, high vibe energy.

Journaling

Journaling is another practice that I knew was good for me, but I struggled to get into. I would buy pretty notebooks and pastel pens with the intention of writing every day, but I would always save it until night time when I ended up being too tired and lazy...I would tell myself that I would write the next morning, but then I wouldn't have time between making my green smoothie and doing some yoga stretches before class...and the cycle continues. I finally committed to journaling every morning for a few minutes and now it has finally stuck! Some days I write half a page, and other days I write seven. Journaling is a therapeutic way to process your emotions and express how you are feeling with words. It is also a time to congratulate yourself on all of your amazing accomplishments from the prior day, which is always fun to look back on if you read through your journal years after the pages have been filled. Putting pen to paper is an amazing way to pause, tap into your head and heart, and take a few moments to care for your soul.

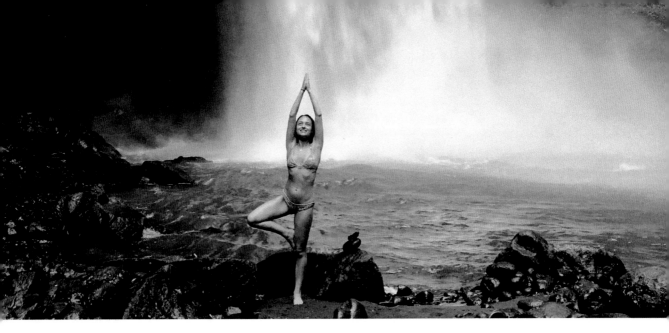

Sloane Elizabeth

Mantras

Stating your intentions or beliefs (either in your head or out loud) is a super powerful way to get your message out into the Universe. Mantras can be "I am" statements, such as "I am loved; I am healthy," or statements about other energies – "The universe has my back; My inner light shines and reaches those around me." There is no "right" way to create or recite a mantra. They also don't have to be limited to ideas that have already come to fruition – for example, your mantra during exam week could be "I am getting A's on all of my exams" even if you haven't taken any yet. In fact, by setting clear intentions and saying these statements aloud, you are taking a step one step closer to achieving everything that you desire. Don't think too hard about your mantras, and don't feel stuck reciting the same statements every day. Mix it up based on what you need to hear in the moment and what your current intentions, hopes, and dreams are.

Visualization/Manifestation

Take a few minutes right now to close your eyes. Using your imagination, create the world you desire. Look around and observe the life that you want to live. Focus on how you FEEL in this life, not necessarily on the exact outcomes. By visualizing situations that you wish to occur while focusing on the feelings associated with this scenario, you are putting the request out into the Universe, and it will respond. If you try to manifest $1 million one day, don't expect to win the lottery the next day. Rather, visualize yourself having financial freedom and pursuing all of the opportunities that would grant you. Tap into how you would feel having these opportunities...then wait and see how the Universe starts giving you little tastes of these experiences and feelings.

Essential Oils

Essential oils come from pressing plants and extracting very pure oil. These are super powerful with many medicinal properties. Essential oils can be used in a diffuser, for aromatherapy, topically, or mixed into drinks. If you are using them for any medicinal purpose, consult a doctor and do research to make sure you don't harm your skin or body. The simplest way to get into essential oils is to buy a starter pack of popular, multi-purpose oils and diffuse them in your room. See how different oils make you feel! Some are shown to improve migraines, brighten your mood, reduce anxiety, or help you sleep. You can also purchase blends of oils that are made for a specific purpose (i.e. enhancing focus).

Keep it simple at first, and experiment with your favorite scents.

Nature

Many people feel grounded and calm in nature. I personally love the intoxicating feeling of the wind in my hair while jetting across a lake at 5 p.m. on a summer day, or hiking along an ocean-side trail until summiting at a beautiful vista outlook. When I don't have access to lakes or mountain tops (i.e. at school in land-locked Nashville), I try to take walks, alone or with friends, and pop on some music. Looking up from my phone, and appreciating the world around me are amazing ways to ground myself, clear my head, and get a fresh perspective.

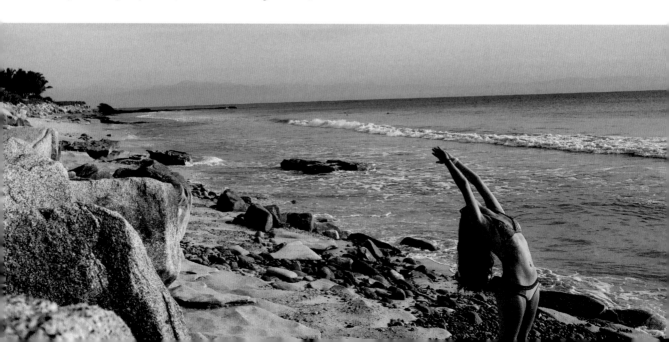

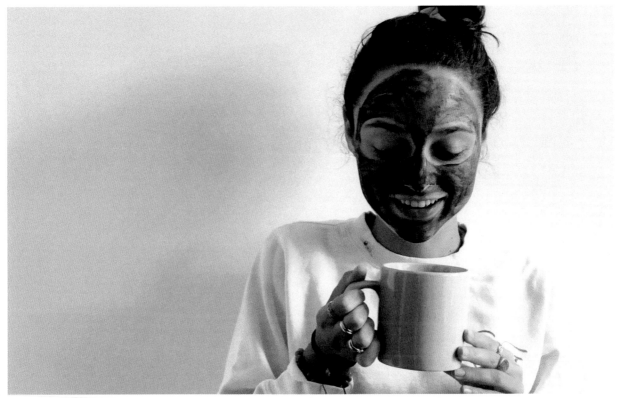

Sloane Elizabeth

Dry brushing

Dry brushes can be bought online or at health food stores – they look like hairbrushes but for your body! They are super easy to use and very beneficial! Before showering, brush your whole body in short strokes towards your heart. Starting at your non-dominant foot, use the brush to make upward strokes. For your arms and neck, brush downward to your heart. This brushing stimulates your lymphatic system, which aids in detoxification and eliminating waste. It may feel a little painful or rough on your skin at first, so be gentle. You should feel good and awake afterwards, and your skin will tingle a bit!

Tea

Drinking herbal tea has so many benefits – it helps you unwind after your day, it may keep you from unnecessary snacking or sugar cravings, and it has great medicinal powers. Making and enjoying a cup of tea after dinner is a super simple self-care practice that I do daily, and it is one of my favorite ways to wrap up my day.

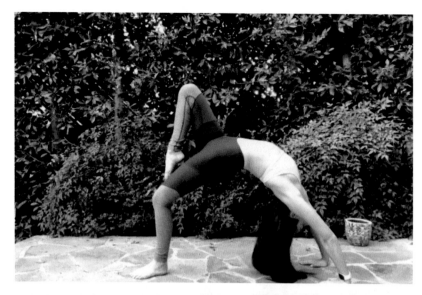

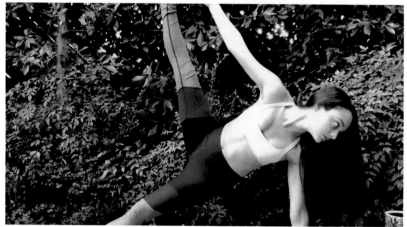

EXERCISE

Of course, being physically active is a key component to leading a healthy life. That being said, you do not need to run a marathon, lift heavy weights, play sports every day, or be an experienced yogi to be physically fit and active! No matter what your fitness goals are, exercise should be a part of your wellness routine. Physical activity is beneficial for your heart, bones, muscles, and mind, and it has been shown to help prevent many chronic diseases.

If you hate going to the gym, then don't go to the gym! There are countless ways that you can exercise, so try different activities and see what works for you. I personally love mixing up my workouts – it keeps your mind interested, and surprising your body with new forms of movements is the best way to continuously challenge yourself and improve your fitness. If you do the same workout every day, then you will likely get tired of it and/or feel like you have plateaued...then again, if you find that you only like one type of workout, then DO it!

Many people (especially girls) are also scared of bulking up, so they only stick to cardio. I believe that cardio, strength training, toning, and stretching should ALL be incorporated into a balanced workout regiment. Having strong, lean, powerful muscles feels so much better and more rewarding than a frail, skinny, exhausted body forced to run on the treadmill for hours every day. Working out should make you feel strong, empowered, and amazing! Especially because endorphins in your brain are released when you workout, you will probably leave your workout feeling happier and clearer minded than when you started!

Another obstacle that many college students run into is time - everyone is constantly busy or tired, and working out easily gets pushed to the bottom of your to-do list. Sometimes, it is absolutely necessary to spend your hour break taking a nap instead of going to a workout class. Other times, getting yourself up and dressed in your fitness gear is exactly what you need to reboot, pump up the energy, and de-stress. Finding the time to move every single day (even if it's only for 20 minutes) will help you stay focused, feel your best, increase your energy, and keep your stress levels low

– all things that will help immeasurably in your college career!

Of course, every body is different. Different forms of movement feel better for some people than others. Working out at the gym three days a week may feel great for one person, while another person thrives on a daily 5 mile run. The most important thing to remember is to listen to YOUR body. Take a rest day when you need it. Push yourself on your sprint times when you're up for it. Set goals for yourself, but don't beat yourself up if you come up short. Find what works for you, and stick to it!

You may feel intimidated walking into your college (or neighborhood) gym - there are tons of machines, weights, and PEOPLE! My recommendations for starting your workout routine if you have never had one before are:

1. Go with a friend!
Try some exercises together, laugh about your lack of knowledge on all of the equipment, and have fun!

2. Use YouTube!
There are hundreds of awesome workout videos online for free. This is my favorite thing to do when I can't make it to a workout class. Having a voice tell you what to do ensures that you are focused and efficient

Sloane Elizabeth

with your time. It also takes away the stress of creating your own series of moves, which can take some time and creativity.

3. Try a workout class at your school gym or off campus!

I am a huge fan of classes – I feel encouraged, challenged, and empowered when I am sweating and working hard in the company of others. I also push myself more when an instructor is telling me what to do. Getting off campus can sometimes be a hassle, so I also recommend trying out free classes that your school gym may offer.

Kale & Kravings

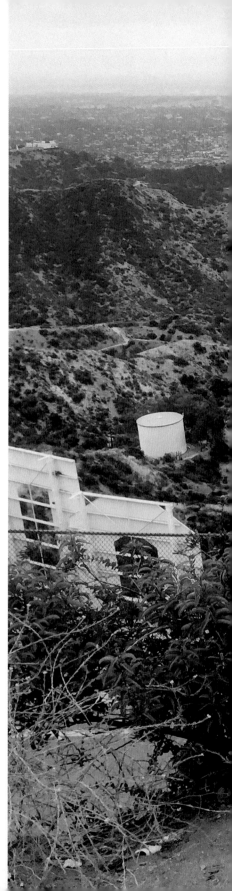

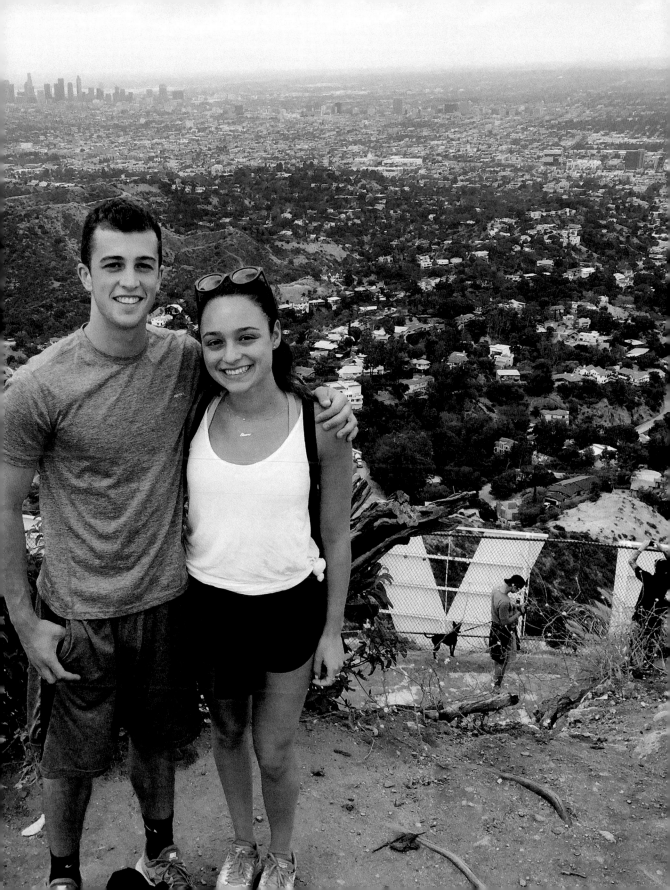

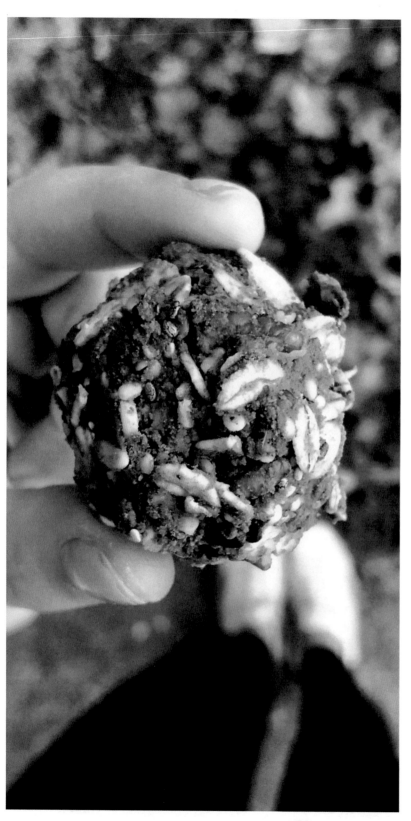

SNACK RECIPES

Sweet Potato Bowl:

Ingredients:

-1 Small sweet potato

-¼ Tsp cinnamon

-½ Tsp coconut butter

-½ Cup dairy free yogurt

-1 Tbsp nut butter

-1 Tsbp chia seeds

-Optional toppings: berries, figs, banana, bee pollen, coconut flakes, granola

Directions:

-Wrap the sweet potato in a damp paper towel and microwave for 4 minutes.

-Flip the sweet potato and microwave for an additional 2-4 minutes (until very soft).

-Peel the potato (or leave the skin on) and mash it in a bowl with the cinnamon and coconut butter.

-Add the rest of the ingredients to the bowl and add optional toppings.

Sloane Elizabeth

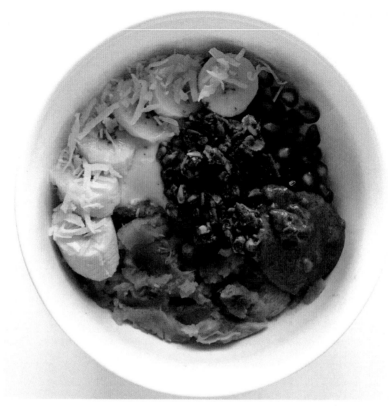

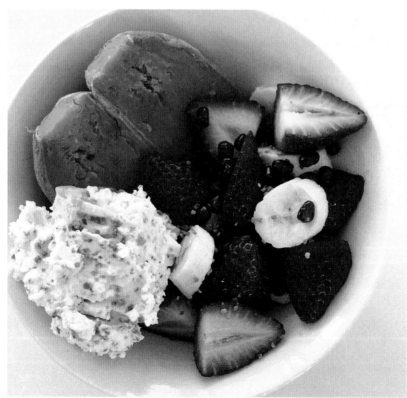

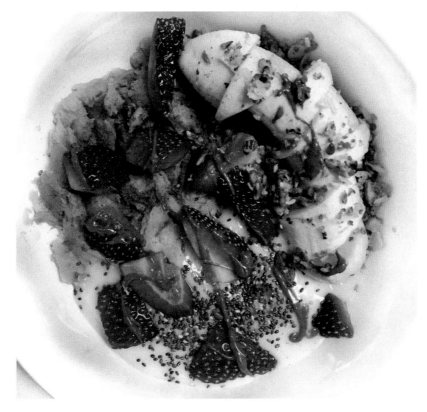

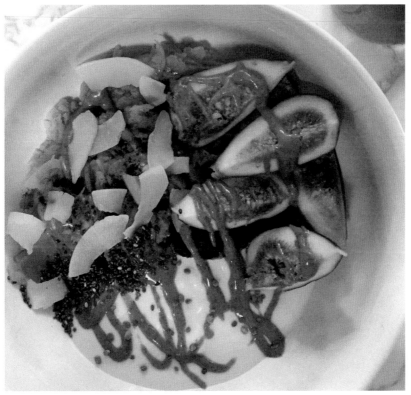

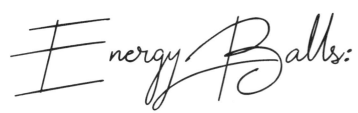

Energy Balls:

(each recipe makes ~12 balls)

Pumpkin Spice
Ingredients:

-¾ Cup rolled oats

-1/3 Cup pumpkin

-¼ Cup almond butter

-1 Tbsp chia seeds

-1 Tbsp flax seeds

-1 Tbsp maca

-2 Scoops vanilla protein

-2 Tbsp cacao nibs

-¼ Tsp cinnamon

-1/2 Tsp pumpkin spice

Chocolate Almond Fudge
Ingredients:

-½ Cup rolled oats

-1 Tbsp cocoa powder

-2 Scoops chocolate protein

-1 Tbsp chia seeds

-¼ Cup unsweetened coconut shreds

-¼ Cup crushed walnuts

-½ Cup almond butter

-2 Tbsp almond milk

-¼ Tsp cinnamon

Chocolate PB
Ingredients:

-1 Cup rolled oats

-2 Scoops chocolate protein

-1 Tbsp chia seeds

-Cinnamon

-1 Tbsp cocoa powder

-¼ Cup coconut flakes

-2 Tbsp crunchy PB

-¼ Cup almond milk

-2 Tbsp cacao nibs

Matcha Spirulina
Ingredients:

-½ Cup oats

-1/3 Cup shredded coconut

-2 Tbsp melted coconut butter

-1 Tbsp mathca powder

-3 Tbsp chia seeds

-2 Scoops vanilla protein powder

-¼ Cup chopped cashews

-1/3 Cup unsweetened almond milk

Directions for all:
Put all of the ingredients in a bowl. Mix with a spoon or your hands. Roll into balls and store in the refrigerator for up to 5 days.

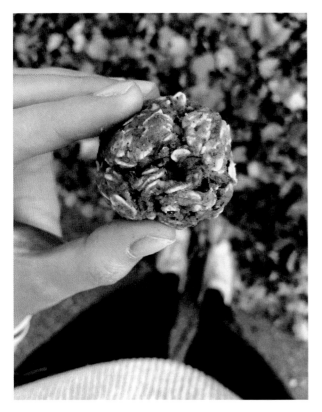
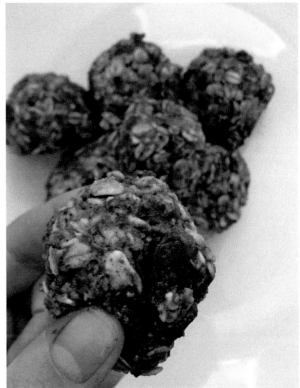

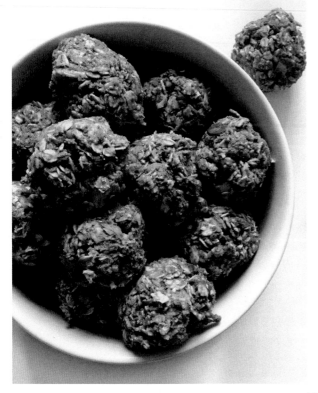
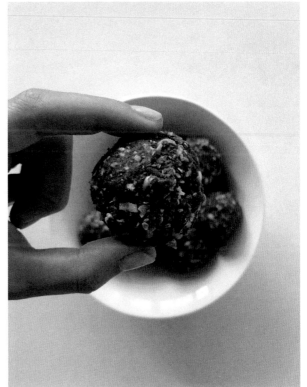

Smoothies:

Berry
Ingredients:
- ½ Frozen banana
- ¼ Cup berries – blueberries, strawberries, raspberries, blackberries
- ½ Cup cauliflower, steamed then frozen
- 1 Tbsp peanut butter
- 1 Scoop vanilla protein
- 1 Tsp acai powder
- ¼ Tsp cinnamon
- Unsweetened almond milk to blend

Strawberry Shortcake
Ingredients:
- ½ Cup cauliflower, steamed then frozen
- ¼ Cup frozen strawberries
- 1 Scoop vanilla protein powder
- ¼ Tsp cinnamon
- 2 Tsp shredded coconut
- 1 Tbsp goji berries
- 1 Tbsp almond butter
- ¼ Avocado
- Unsweetened almond milk to blend

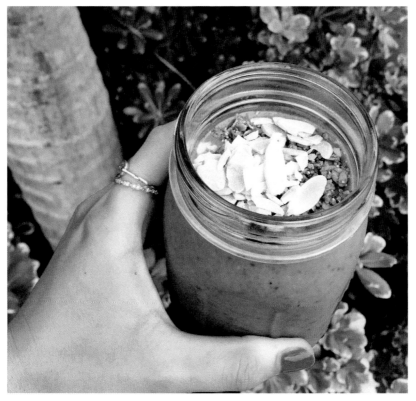

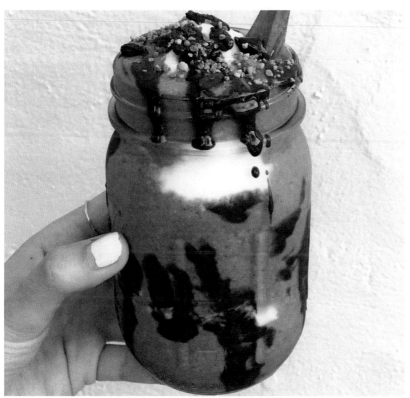

Smoothies:

Peanut Butter Chocolate
Ingredients:

-½ Frozen banana

-½ Cup zucchini, steamed then frozen

-1 Scoop chocolate protein

-1 Tbsp cacao powder

-1 Tbsp cacao nibs

-1 Tbsp hemp seeds

-2 Tbsp peanut butter

-Unsweetened almond milk to blend

Sweet Potato Pie
Ingredients:

-½ Sweet potato, steamed then frozen

-½ Cup cauliflower, steamed then frozen

-1 Tsp cinnamon

-¼ Tsp nutmeg

-¼ Tsp vanilla extract

-1 Tbsp chia seeds

-1 Scoop vanilla protein powder

-2 Tbsp almond butter

-Unsweetened almond milk to blend

Mint Chip
Ingredients:

-½ Banana

-1 Cup spinach

-1 Scoop vanilla protein

-Handful of fresh mind leaves

-2 Tbsp cacao nibs

-¼ Avocado

-1 Tbsp coconut oil

-1 Tbsp flax seeds

-Unsweetened almond milk to blend

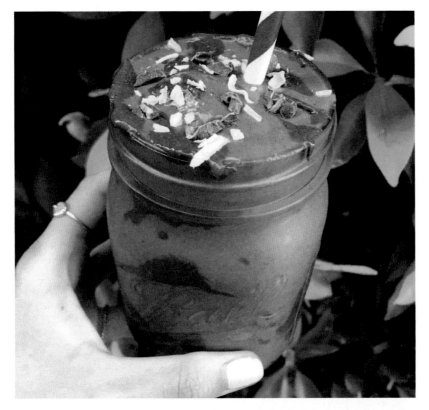

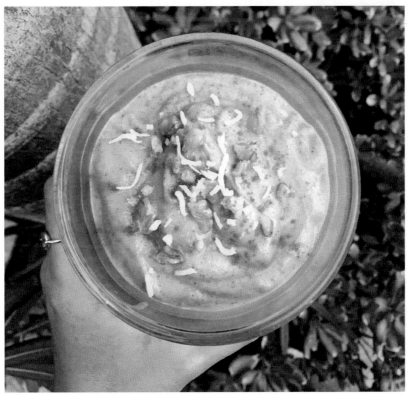

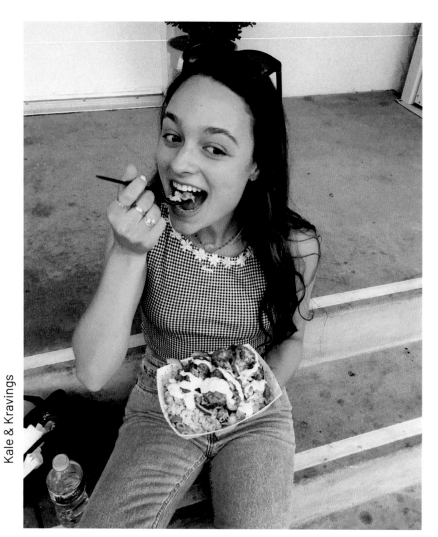

INTUITIVE EATING

Eat when you are hungry; stop when you are full. Sounds easy, right? Then why can it be so hard?! Intuitive eating is the practice of using your intuition (i.e. listening to your body's feelings) to guide your eating practices. There are many factors that may influence what your body is trying to tell you...the purely physical aspect of this being hunger. Does your stomach want food? Or is your stomach full? If we have been ignoring our hunger signs and simply eat because it is "lunch time," or we overeat because the food just tastes SO good, then it may be hard to actually identify whether or not we are truly hungry. A couple of ways to work on this:

1. Actually stop and THINK about how you are feeling!

After you've been practicing intuitive eating for a while, you may not need to take this conscious step. However, this active thought is probably necessary when you are first starting out. Do a scan of your body and assess how it feels physically.

2. Drink a glass of water!

Sometimes we feel hungry because we are dehydrated. Aim to drink water throughout the day to avoid this bodily confusion.

3. Use a hunger scale!

This is something that I learned in a podcast that I use with a lot of my clients... -10 is absolutely empty, depleted, near death hunger and +10 is stuffed to the brim, probably throwing up because you ate so much. The aim of the game is to stay between a -3 and +3. By checking in with your body before, during, and after you eat using this scale, you can more easily assess your level of hunger. If you finish a meal and feel like a +1, wait 20 minutes, and then decide if you want more food to bring yourself closer to a +3. Our bodies need time to digest and process the fact that we have eaten food, so take some time between helpings if you are considering going for seconds.

Intuitive eating is not just about physical hunger though; it is also about listening to your body when choosing WHAT to eat. This has three prongs as well – the physical, the mental, and the emotional.

Physically speaking, you may experience certain ailments or symptoms if you are deficient in a certain nutrient (i.e. bruising and anemia if you are low on iron, weakness and dizziness if you are low on sugar). Feeding yourself food that makes your body feel good, nourished, and strong is a key part of the health and wellness puzzle.

Food is not just about the chemical nutrients and macro building blocks though. As humans, we have taste preferences, favorite foods, and cravings! Being intuitive and true to yourself means honoring those cravings and preferences. Don't like kale? Don't eat it! Love chocolate? Find ways to incorporate it into your smoothies and desserts! Some people may think...."ok so intuitive eating means that I can eat my favorite McDonald's meal every day because it makes me happy??" Not exactly ...eating McDonald's probably doesn't make your body feel great, if we're being real. If it makes your heart happy, then maybe treat yourself every so often! Once you embrace a healthy lifestyle, the foods that you crave and intuitively want WILL BE healthy, nutritious, delicious, and nourishing for you body, mind, and soul.

Emotional eating happens for everyone. Feeling sad may make you crave homemade brownies with tons of ice cream, or a warm

bowl of macaroni and cheese. Winter weather is a cue for hot chocolate and peppermint mochas. Christmas dinner brings back memories of buttery mashed potatoes and roasted ham. When it comes to emotions, honor them – feeding your soul should not be shameful. We are human beings, and we are not meant to eat perfectly "clean, healthy" diets 24/7! Where's the fun in that?! One form of emotional eating that can be especially tricky for college students is stress eating. This often occurs during exam time when you are tired, stressed, dehydrated, busy, and all you want is junk food and sugar! Sound familiar?? When our bodies are put into this physical state, our brains want simple sugars that will metabolize quickly and give us energy FAST. While a bag of m&m's and a venti iced vanilla latte might make you feel better for an hour, you will likely feel a major crash right when you're getting back into productive study mode. If you find yourself in this stressed out,
hangry mood:

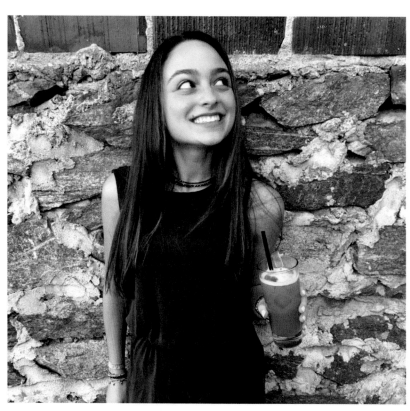

1. Assess if you are actually hungry or just tired.

If you are actually hungry, aim for a snack that has complex carbs + protein/fat. Your body needs sustenance and good energy, not just sugar! If you are NOT hungry but still need something to munch on, make some herbal tea and snack on fruits and veggies that have a high water content – celery, cucumber, watermelon. This will keep you occupied without feeling stuffed and bloated.

2. Take a few deep breaths!

The power of deep breathing is SO strong. Taking just 30 seconds to decompress can be the perfect study break to relax, de-stress, and refocus. Even if you don't practice yoga, I'm sure you can figure out how to take some nice, deep yogi breaths.

3. Move!

Our bodies are not meant to sit at a desk for hours on end. If you have a lot of studying to do, get up and do some jumping jacks or yoga stretches every hour. Try moving locations every few hours, or even just choose a new desk in the library! You'll feel refreshed once you move away from the stagnant energy created from hours of studying in the same position.

Intuitive eating seems really easy, and it may be for some people, but for many others it can be really hard and confusing! There are tons of online resources and books to help you get more in tune with your body. Remember to experiment, trust yourself, and don't compare your hunger and body to another person's. YOU are unique, and that is so freaking cool!!

Sloane Elizabeth

Kale & Kravings

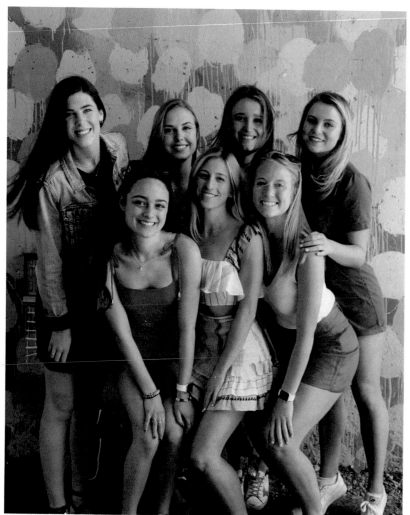

TRIPS

Some of the most fun college experiences I've had have been on weekend trips with my friends! I've been on many 10+ hour long road trips in my college career, and, of course, I am always the one people look to for SNACKS! Travelling while maintaining a healthy diet and lifestyle can be tricky, no matter where you are going. For people who like routine, a new environment without your normal food/kitchen/gym can be a source of anxiety. However, trips are meant to be FUN!

So here are my top tips for enjoying amazing adventures and travels while in college...

1. Be prepared with snacks!

I'm the girl who brought an entire suitcase filled with food to college (anyone surprised?!), and you are guaranteed to see me with 1-2 grocery bags filled with snacks for any weekend trip my friends and I take! Many times, I know I won't have a place to refrigerate food on the trip, so I resort to healthy snack foods.

Here is my go to list:

-Rice cakes

-Nut butters

-Bananas, apples, oranges, avocados, lemons (non-refrigerated fruits)

-Homemade energy balls

-Veggie chips (kale, beets)

-Oatmeal packets

-Gluten-free pretzels

-Protein bars

-Trail mix/mixed nuts

-Coconut water

2. Bring as many of your regular foods as you can!

I always bring my supplements and some tea no matter where I go. Having even a small piece of your normal routine ensures that your body still feels as good as possible while you're out exploring and having fun with your friends!

3. Stay active!

Rarely do I go to a hotel gym or a workout class when I'm in a different city. Instead, I try to walk, bike, or hike wherever I am. There are so many ways to stay active while away from home, so try to keep your body moving.

4. Live in the moment and let go!

While many of my college trips have been amazingly fun, they have not been my healthiest days...alcohol is usually involved (in copious amounts for many people), sleep is rarely a priority, and I usually arrive back at school completely exhausted. In these moments, I always remind myself to let go and remember that this is COLLEGE! These will be the craziest, wildest, most fun times of our lives. I would much rather remember a trip for the amazing memories than for my anxiety over where I could find an avocado or apple cider vinegar. With that being said, know your limits and what you can handle. Everyone's emotional, alcohol, and food tolerances are different, so look out for yourself and honor your body.

Sloane Elizabeth

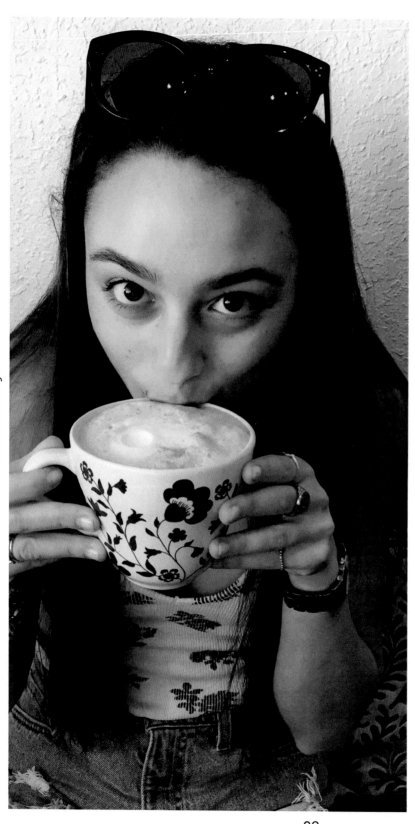

DRINK & SAUCE RECIPES

Turmeric Latte:

Ingredients:

-1 Cup unsweetened almond milk

-1 Tbsp ground turmeric powder

-1 Tsp ground ginger powder

-1 Tsp cinnamon

-1 Tsp coconut oil

-1/8 Tsp black pepper

-1 Tsp honey

Directions:

-Heat almond milk in the microwave for 2-3 minutes.

-Add the rest of the ingredients and whisk together (or combine in a blend for 20 seconds).

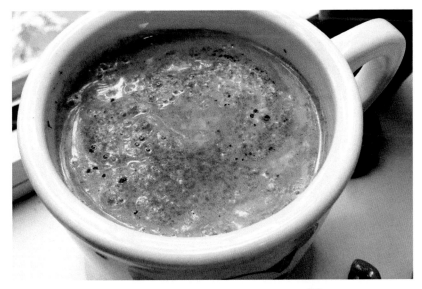

Super Matcha Latte:

Ingredients:
- ½ Cup water
- 1 Tsp matcha powder
- ¼ Tsp cinnamon
- 1 Tsp coconut butter
- ½ Tsp maca powder
- 1 Scoop collagen
- ½ Tsp honey (optional)
- ½ Cup unsweetened almond milk

Directions:
-Heat water in the microwavefor 2-3 minutes.
-Add the rest of theingredients and whisk to-
gether (or combine in a blend for 20 seconds).

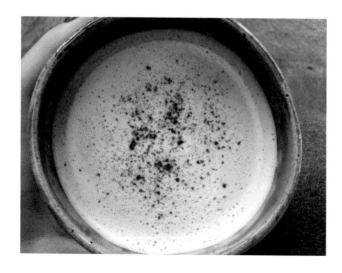

Healthy Hot Cocoa:

Ingredients:
-1 Cup unsweetened almond milk
-2 Tbsp cocoa powder
-¼ Tsp cinnamon
-¼ Tsp vanilla extract
-1/2 Tsp honey

Directions:
-Heat almond milk in the microwave for 2-3 minutes.
-Add the rest of the ingredients and whisk together (or combine in a blend for 20 seconds).

Morning Drink:

Ingredients:
-1 Cup warm water
-Juice from ½ lemon
-½ Tsp ground turmeric
-½ Tsp ground ginger
-1/8 Tsp cayenne pepper
-1/8 Tsp black pepper

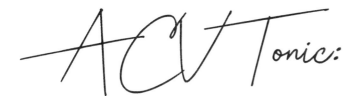

ACV Tonic:

Ingredients:

- 1 Cup cold water
- 1/2 Tbsp apple cider vinegar
- 1/8 Tsp cayenne pepper
- ¼ Tsp ground ginger powder

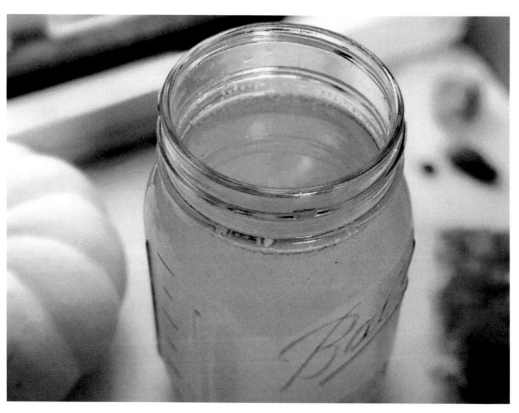

Vegan Pesto:

(2 servings)

Ingredients:
- 1/3 Cup raw cashews
- ¼ Cup kale
- 1/3 Cup broccoli
- 2 Cloves of garlic
- 2 Tbsp nutritional yeast
- ¼ Avocado
- Juice from 1 lemon
- Zest from ½ lemon
- 2 Tbsp olive oil
- Black pepper + pink sea salt

Directions:
- Soak cashews in water for atleast 6 hours.
- Blend all of the ingredients together.

Sloane Elizabeth

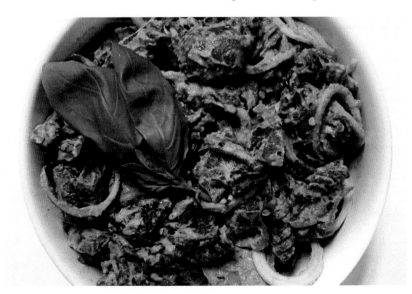

Vegan Cheeze Sauce:

Ingredients:

-1/3 Cup butternut squash

-1 Tsp dijon mustard

-1/3 Cup raw cashews

-1 Tbsp nutritional yeast

-¼ Tsp onion powder

-1 Clove garlic

-Juice from ½ lemon

-Black pepper + pink sea salt

-Water (or unsweetened almond milk) to blend

Directions:

-Soak the cashews in water for at least 6 hours.

-Put the butternut squash in a microwave-safe bowel with 2 tbsp water.

-Cover the bowl with a damp paper towel and microwave for ~4 minutes until cooked thoroughly.

-Rinse the cashews. Add all of the ingredients to a blender.

-Blend until creamy.

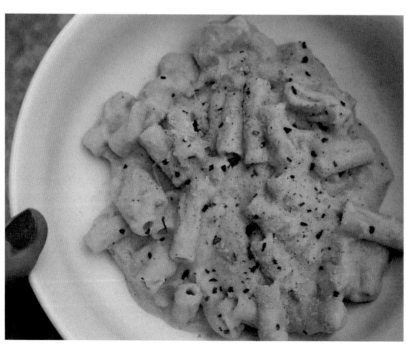

Zucchini Alfredo Sauce:

Ingredients:

-1 Large zucchini

-1/3 Cup raw cashews

-1 Glove garlic

-Juice from ¼ lemon

-¼ Cup full fat coconut cream

-Black pepper + pink sea salt

Directions:

-Soak the cashews in water for at least 6 hours.

-Slice the zucchini into disks and place in a microwave safe bowl. Cover with a damp paper towel and microwave for 3 minutes.

-Rinse the cashews. Add all of the ingredients to a blender.

-Blend until creamy.

Sloane Elizabeth

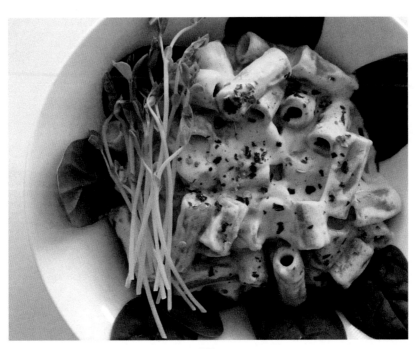

Lemon Tahini Dressing:

Ingredients:

-Juice from ½ lemon

-1 Tbsp tahini

-1 Tbsp Dijon mustard

-Black pepper + pink sea salt

Directions:

-Whisk all of the ingredients together and use on salads and bowls.

-Blend until creamy.

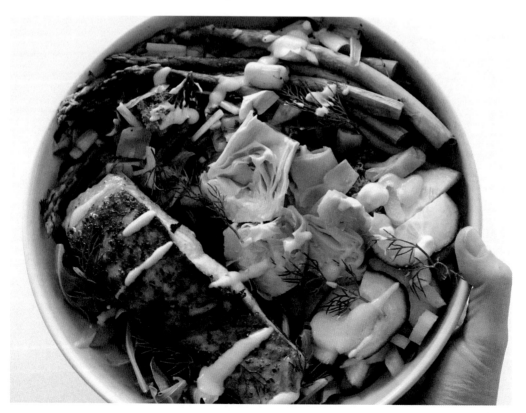

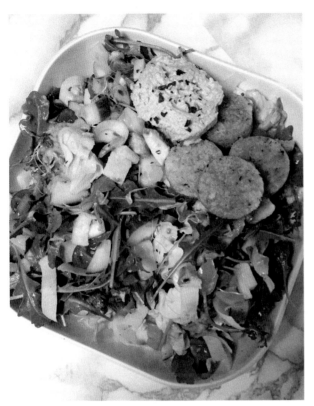
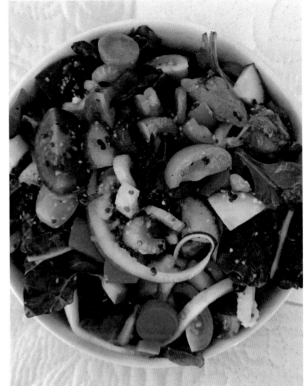

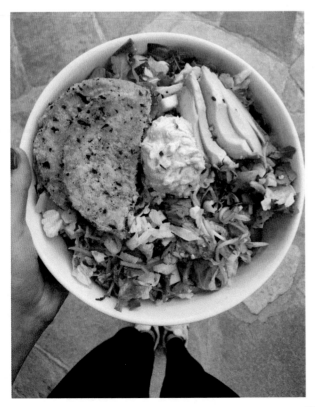
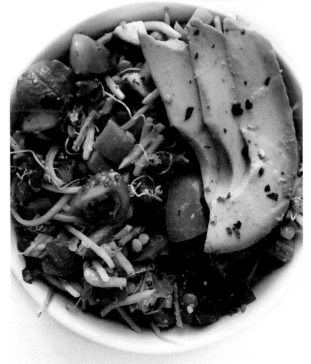

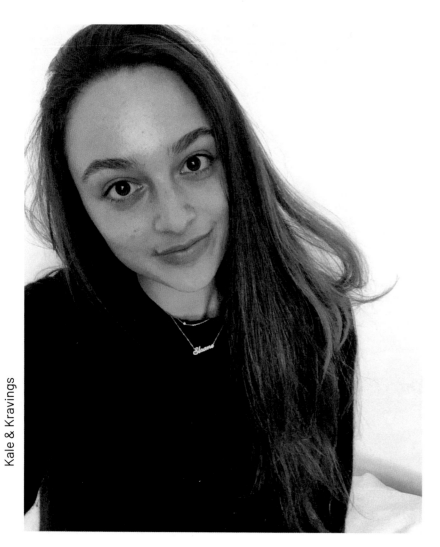

Kale & Kravings

IMMUNE SYSTEM

Being in college is amazing because you get to live with other college students! I have absolutely loved being able to hang out with friends essentially 24/7. The downside of having tons of people living in very close proximity to one another is sickness. Many other factors contribute to the colds, flus, and coughs that tend to sweep college campuses – lack of sleep, stress, poor eating, sharing cups/utensils...the list goes on. Caring for your immune system will be a tremendous help to you when everyone starts getting sick just around exam time! Here are some tips for keeping your white blood cells happy and strong:

1. Get enough sleep!
I will continue to say this a million times... please sleep!!! Sleep is your body's time to restore itself and rest (not to mention process all of the flash cards you just tried to cram into your brain for tomorrow's quiz!).

When you are rundown and sleep deprived, your immune system is compromised and will not be able to help protect you from germs as effectively.

2. Drink tons of water!
Water helps to flush out all of the toxins in your body. If you are constantly dehydrated, those toxins get to hang out in your body and grow until they make you sick! Yuck!

3. Load up on vitamin C!
Many foods are amazing sources of this essential vitamin, so try to get these into your diet on a daily basis. If you don't have access to these, a supplement will work too.

4. Consume probiotics!
Probiotics are good bacteria that help keep your gut working well. The health of your intestines is SUPER important for your overall immune system – when there are lots of good bacteria in your system, there is physically less surface area available for bad bacteria. Probiotic-rich foods include sauerkraut, kimchi, kombucha, kefir, and

yogurt. A good supplement is also a great idea to incorporate into your daily wellness regiment.

5. Relax!
Stress is another factor that harms your immune system. By incorporating self-care regiments and practices like yoga, meditation, deep breathing, and laughing into your day, you are helping your mind relax and your body strengthen its immune response – win, win!

-Oranges
-Strawberries
-Pineapple
-Mango
-Brussel
Sprouts

-Kiwi
-Red bell peppers
-Broccoli
-Kale
-Papaya
-Cauliflower

Sloane Elizabeth

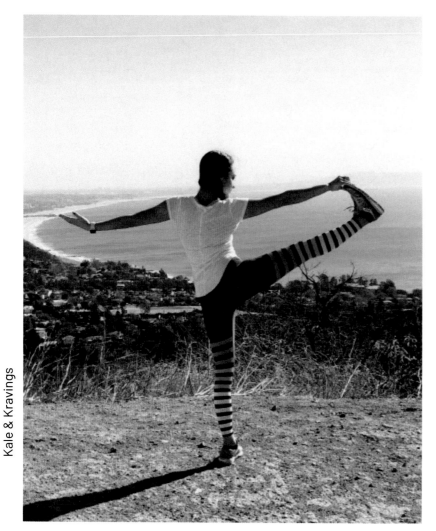

ROUTINE

All of the topics in this book are incredibly valuable and unique to YOU! The best way to find a healthy lifestyle for yourself is to be patient, experiment, and stay in tune with your body. Once you've found what works for you, establishing a steady routine will help keep you on track and feeling your best! I love having a morning routine – I do the same set of activities almost every morning. I look forward to my mornings (I never thought I would be able to say that

I'm a morning person!), and I am able to start my day on an amazing note. Having a routine is also helpful for when you are moving or traveling. Grounding yourself in familiar behaviors makes the transition much smoother, and you are much less likely to deviate from your health and wellness habits! Remember, don't compare your routine to your friends'…what you do every day should make YOU happy and feel good to YOU, and that is all that matters.

Find your groove and stick to it, but remember to spice it up from time to time too!

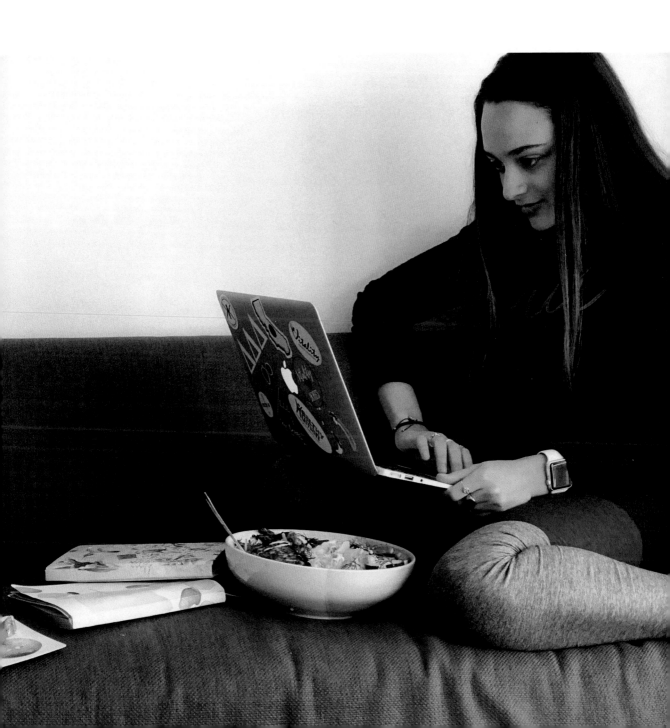

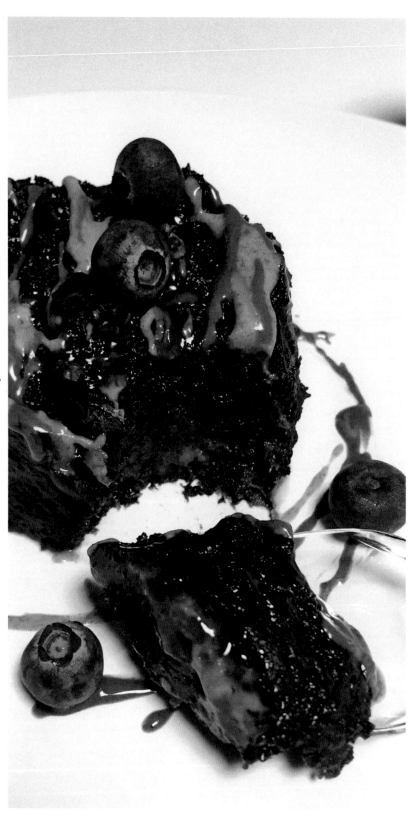

DESSERT RECIPES

Chocolate Lava Mug Cake:

Ingredients:

-1 Ripe banana

-3 Tbsp cacao powder

-2 Tbsp nut butter of choice

-Dash of cinnamon

-Pink of pink salt

-1/8 Tsp baking soda

Directions:

-Mash banana in a bowl.

-Mix in the rest of the ingredients.

-Transfer to a microwave safe mug or bowl.

-Microwave for 2-3 minutes until the cake is cooked almost all the way through (since it is vegan, you can eat it raw/gooey!)

Sloane Elizabeth

Mint Chip Nice Cream:

Ingredients:

-2 Frozen bananas

-Handful of mint leaves

-2 Tbsp cacao nibs

Directions

-Blend all ingredients together.

-Add a bit of water or almond milk if your blender needs it.

-Serve immediately or store in the freezer.

No Bake Vegan Cookie Dough Balls:

Ingredients:
-1 Can chickpeas
-¾ Tsp vanilla extract
-1 Tbsp maple syrup
-2 Dates
-½ Cup almond butter
-¼ Tsp pink salt
-2 Tbsp cacao nibs
-2 Tbsp chocolate chips

Directions:
-Rinse the chickpeas and "de-shell" them (peel off the filmy outer layer).
-Blend all of the ingredients in a blender or food processer (except for the cacao nibs and chocolate chips) until smooth.
-Mix in the chocolates.
-Roll into balls and store in the freezer for at least 1 hour. Enjoy, and store in the refrigerator!

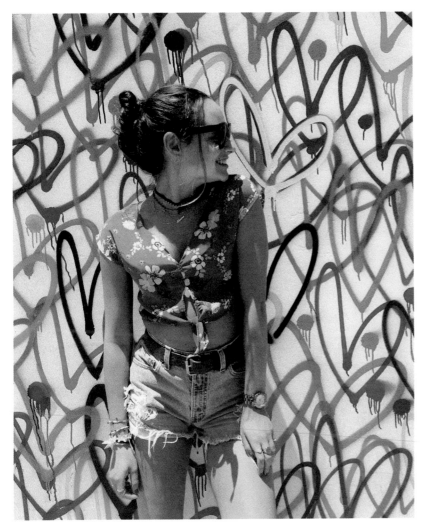

CONCLUSION

Sloane Elizabeth

Health and wellness is a holistic idea. Though scientific, there is not one way to be "healthy." Drinking kale smoothies every day makes me feel great, but it may not work for you. If you feel good, stay in tune with your body, listen to what it is asking you for, stay curious and knowledgeable about your health, and make your wellness a priority, then you are on the right track! I believe that a sustainable, balanced lifestyle feels best to most people. When you are following a way of life instead of strict rules and lists of "good" and "bad" foods, you will never "mess up!" That is the Kale & Kravings approach. College is an amazing and exciting, yet weird and difficult time, and finding the balance between fun and fitness, partying and prepping meals, and studying and sleep is what it's all about. For some, this balance comes naturally; for everyone else, there's Kale & Kravings.

56855861R00049

Made in the USA
Middletown, DE
24 July 2019